D0534071

BASIC ATHLETIC TRAINING

An Introductory Course in the Care and Prevention of Athletic Injuries

6th ed.

Ken Wright, D.A., ATC

Scott Barker, M.S., ATC

Jason Bennett, D.A., ATC

Randy Deere, D.A., AT-R

in cooperation with

Cramer Products, Inc
www.cramersportsmed.com

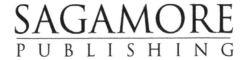

SAGAMORE PUBLISHING

©2013 Sagamore Publishing LLC
All rights reserved.

Publishers: Joseph J. Bannon and Peter L. Bannon
Director of Sales and Marketing: William A. Anderson
Marketing Coordinator: Emily Wakefield
Director of Development and Production: Susan M. Davis
Technology Manager: Christopher Thompson
Production Coordinator: Amy S. Dagit
Cover Designer: Reata Strickland

ISBN print edition: 978-1-57167-759-4
ISBN ebook: 978-1-57167- 760-0
LCCN: 2013941501

SAGAMORE
PUBLISHING

1807 N. Federal Dr.
Urbana, IL 61801
www.sagamorepub.com

The authors, along with all contributors to the manual, would like to dedicate this text to all the young professionals in the discipline of athletic training.

Preface

Basic Athletic Training, 6th edition, is written and edited by certified athletic trainers and a physician as a comprehensive introduction to current philosophies, procedures and practices related to the care and prevention of athletic injuries. Designed as a classroom textbook, *Basic Athletic Training* will prove to be challenging and rewarding for the athletic training student. It also serves as a reference guide for individuals concerned with the health and well-being of athletes. This text is divided into 13 chapters and provides the reader with a step-by-step presentation of various duties and responsibilities utilized by physicians, athletic trainers, and other licensed healthcare provider. With web-based educational videos and materials on selected anatomical content, Chapters 6-12 are devoted to exploration of various body structures and how to prevent, evaluate, and treat injuries that might be associated with these structures. The web-based educational videos and materials allow the student to view dynamic aspects of joint anatomy (bones, ligaments, muscles), dermatomes and myotomes, basic treatment protocol, evaluation format, common injuries, and referral guidelines. The sections within the Appendix will help the athletic training student become familiar with common words (root word, prefixes, and suffixes), a glossary of terms, and websites for health care and sport industry professionals. At the completion of the text, the athletic training student will have learned the basics of athletic training and have a working knowledge of common preventive, evaluation, treatment, and rehabilitation techniques in sports medicine. Through this knowledge, the athletic training student will be better prepared to assist the physician and other licensed healthcare provider in caring for athletes and other physically active individuals.

Special Thanks

The authors would like to thank Sagamore Publishing, LLC for providing the financial support for this project. Without their support, we would not have been able to complete the 6th edition of *Basic Athletic Training*. The authors would also like to thank the following individuals for their assistance in the development of this manual: Ms. Reata Strickland as cover designer; Dr. Vivian Wright for her expertise; Ms. Whitney Larsen, Ms. Kelly Wright, and Ms. Kendra Wright for serving as guest reviewers, and Ms. Page Love for her expertise.

Acknowledgments

The authors are extremely grateful to the following for their meticulous review, comments, and contributions during the development and update of this book:

- Wayne Bush, M.D., FACS, Western Kentucky University, Bowling Green, KY
- Rodney Brown, M.A., LAT, ATC, The University of Alabama, Tuscaloosa, AL
- Katy Curran Casey, M.S., ATC, CSCS Centers for Disease Control and Prevention, Atlanta, GA
- Fred Hina, M.A., ATC, University of Louisville, Louisville, KY
- Timothy Neal, M.S., ATC, Syracuse University, Syracuse, NY
- Ron H. Walker, M.A., LAT, ATC, CSCS, The University of Tulsa, Tulsa, OK
- Katherine Wright, PT, D.P.T., M.S., Memorial Hermann Sports Medicine, Houston, TX

Basic Athletic Training, *6th ed.*

Contents

About the Authors

Ken Wright, D.A., ATC

Dr. Ken Wright is a professor and director of the Sport Management Program at The University of Alabama. Dr. Wright received his doctor of arts degree from Middle Tennessee State University (1984), master of science degree from Syracuse University (1976), and bachelor of science degree from Eastern Kentucky University (1974). He has served as head athletic trainer at the University of North Carolina at Charlotte and Morehead State University and assistant athletic trainer at Ohio University. Additionally, he was selected as Outstanding Alumnus at Eastern Kentucky University (2001), and he received the Academic Excellence Award from The University of Alabama. In 2012, Dr. Wright was appointed as a member of the board of directors of the United States Anti-Doping Agency. Since 1990, he has served as a Doping Control Officer during which time he worked three Olympic Games (London, Vancouver, and Salt Lake City). Ken has been involved with the United States Olympic Committee as an athletic trainer, educator, and invited presenter at numerous sports medicine and sport management meetings in China, Japan, United Kingdom, Canada, and the United States. From the National Athletic Trainers' Association, Dr. Wright received the Sayers "Bud" Miller Distinguished Educator of the Year Award (2000), Distinguished Athletic Trainer Award (2006), and Athletic Trainer Service Award (1996). Dr. Wright has numerous publications to his credit, including a series of 13 videos (*Sports Medicine Evaluation* and *Sports Medicine Taping*), a computer-assisted instructional program (*Sports Injuries*), and textbooks (*Basic Athletic Training, Preventive Techniques: Taping/Wrapping Techniques and Protective Devices*, and *The Comprehensive Manual of Taping & Wrapping Techniques*). Additionally, he has served on the editorial board of the *Journal of Athletic Training, Physical Therapy in Sport*, and *Sports Medicine Update*, athletic training education accreditation visits, and various USADA, USOC, and NATA committees.

Scott Barker, M.S., ATC

Scott Barker is the head athletic trainer and adjunct faculty for the graduate athletic training education program at California State University, Chico. He received his master of science degree in exercise and sport sciences with a specialization in athletic training from the University of Arizona (1985) and his bachelor of science degree in physical education from the University of Arizona (1984). Barker served for eight years on the National Athletic Trainers Association Education Council Continuing Education Committee and for nine years on the National Athletic Trainers Association Education Multimedia Committee. During this time, Mr. Barker helped with the inception and development of the National Athletic Trainers' Association Virtual Library (online continuing education courses). Barker has received numerous awards in the area of educational multimedia in athletic training including the 2000, 2001, 2002, 2004, 2005, and 2008 National Athletic Trainers' Association, Educational Multimedia Committee, Educational Software Production Contest ATC Commercial Winner; the 2006 National Athletic Trainers' Association, Educational Multimedia Committee, Educational DVD/Video Production Contest ATC Commercial Winner; the 2006 National Athletic Trainers' Association Continuing Education Excellence Award; and the 2007 MERLOT Classic Award for Exemplary Online Learning Resource. Barker has been an invited presenter at 15 National Athletic Trainers' Association Annual Meeting and Clinical Symposium conferences.

Jason Bennett, D.A., ATC

Jason Bennett is a tenured associate professor and program director of the athletic training education program at Chapman University. He received his doctorate at Middle Tennessee State University and both his bachelor's and master's degrees at California State University, Chico. Prior to becoming the program director, Dr. Bennett was the clinical education coordinator for eight years at Chapman University. Dr. Bennett has more than 18 years experience as a certified athletic trainer in Division I, II and III intercollegiate athletics, as well as in minor league baseball. Along with clinical experience, his research interests include the utilization of instructional technologies to enhance student learning.

Randy Deere, D.A., AT-R

Dr. Randy Deere is a professor and program coordinator for the Graduate Sport Administration Program Athletic Administration Concentration at Western Kentucky University. Dr. Deere received his doctor of arts degree from Middle Tennessee State University in 1992, master of arts degree from Austin Peay State University in 1979, and a bachelor of science degree from Middle Tennessee State University in 1978. Dr. Deere spent 14 years as a collegiate athletic trainer before moving into university teaching. Dr. Deere's research interest focuses on online instructional pedagogy. Dr. Deere received the W. H. Mustaine Distinguished Service Award from the Kentucky Association of Health Physical Education Recreation and Dance (KAHPERD) in 2007, the University PE Teacher of the year award from KAHERD in 1998, and the WKU Faculty Service Award for the College of Health and Human Service in 2004. Dr. Deere has numerous national publications and presentations and served as *KAHPERD Journal* editor from 1993 until 2008. Additionally, Deere has served as a reviewer for Wolters Kluwer/ Lippincott Williams and Wilkins and created the PowerPoint supplements for *Applied Sports Medicine for Coaches* in 2009. He served as a Doping Control Officer for the United States Anti-Doping Agency from 2002 until 2008.

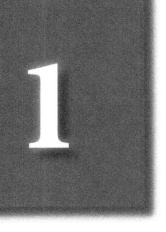

Organization and Administration

Basic Athletic Training 6th ed. is primarily designed for any introductory entry-level (interscholastic or intercollegiate) athletic training student. Additionally, athletic coaches, administrators, student athletes, and their parents can use this book as a resource guide for a better understanding of specific sports-related injuries, emergency procedures, as well as for increasing knowledge about athletic training practices and career opportunities. This edition provides web-based videos and materials, highlighting anatomy, joint range of motion, muscle function, and evaluation formats. It is the goal of this text to stimulate further learning in the identification, treatment/care, and prevention of sports-specific injuries.

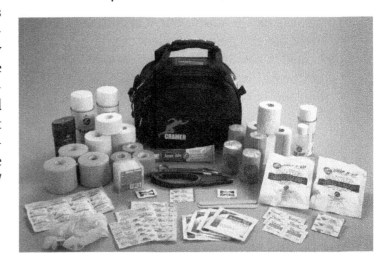

Educational Objectives

Upon completing this chapter, the reader will be able to do the following:
- Identify the competencies of the certified athletic trainer
- Name the duties of the athletic training student
- Identify the members of the sports medicine team and their responsibilities
- Identify the educational programs for athletic training students
- Recognize the National Athletic Trainers' Association (NATA) as the leader in the athletic training allied health care profession
- Describe the fundamental components of an athletic training facility

What is Athletic Training?

Simply stated, athletic training is the prevention, recognition, evaluation, treatment, rehabilitation, and health care administration of athletic injuries. However, implementation of the athletic training concept by a school system is not a simple action, for the program does not begin and end with the person designated as the certified athletic trainer. In fact, the program involves an entire team of people, including not only the certified athletic trainer (ATC), student athletic trainers, student athletes, and team physicians, but also parents, coaches, the equipment manager, school administration, and maintenance personnel.

The certified athletic trainer is a highly educated and skilled professional specializing in health care of the physically active. In cooperation with physicians and other allied health personnel, the certified athletic trainer functions as an integral member of the health care team in sports medicine clinics, industrial settings, professional sports programs, educational institutions, and other athletic health care settings.

National Athletic Trainers' Association

The National Athletic Trainers' Association (NATA) was founded in 1950. It has evolved into a highly respected organization with more than 35,000 members, including over 7,500 student members. The mission of NATA is to enhance the quality of health care provided by certified athletic trainers and to advance the athletic training profession. In 1990, the American Medical Association (AMA) recognized athletic training as an allied health care profession. This endorsement provides monumental benefits for the advancement of athletic training as a profession and for the professional development of the athletic training student. NATA is the primary professional association of athletic trainers in the United States. Since the early 1960s, NATA has assumed the leadership in establishing high standards for the education and certification of athletic trainers. For more information on professional preparation and/or careers in athletic training, please contact:

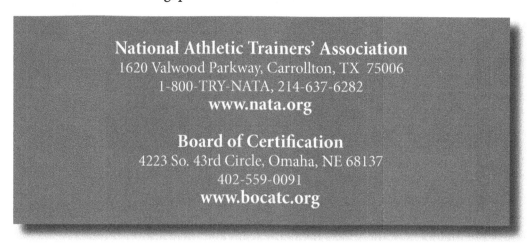

National Athletic Trainers' Association
1620 Valwood Parkway, Carrollton, TX 75006
1-800-TRY-NATA, 214-637-6282
www.nata.org

Board of Certification
4223 So. 43rd Circle, Omaha, NE 68137
402-559-0091
www.bocatc.org

Establishing an Athletic Training/Sports Medicine Program

Checklist for Safety in Sports

To establish an effective athletic training program, school administrators should seek the following:
- A certified athletic trainer (ATC)
- Designated area within the facility for medical care/athletic training room
- Medical files that include accident injury reports, parental consent, insurance referral, and other reports
- Adequate funding to run an effective program
- Educational program for athletes
- Emergency medical action plan
- First aid, wound care, taping and wrapping supplies
- Information regarding confidentiality (FERPA, HIPAA) (The Health Insurance Portability and Accountability Act of 1996) to ensure standards are followed
- Injury notification system

- Medical and dental insurance
- Qualified coaches
- Qualified officials
- Safe sport equipment and facilities
- Require pre-participation physical examinations.
- All coaches, cheerleader, band, and drill team sponsors be certified in cardiopulmonary resuscitation (CPR), automated external defibrillator (AED), American Red Cross Sports Safety Training (SST), and related American Heart Association certifications.

The Sports Medicine Team

The athletic training program starts with the individual appointed to supervise the care and prevention of athletic injuries, a certified athletic trainer or ATC. Before establishing an athletic training room and ordering supplies, the ATC should perform a most important function: finding a team physician. The team physician will provide medical supervision of the ATC and staff members.

Team Physician

The team physician promotes the success of the athletic training program. And, since athletic success is dependent on the health of the players, each team's success could be directly related to the amount of time the physician can devote to the athletic training program. The team physician is the "cornerstone" of the medical team, which should include the certified athletic trainer, coaches, athletic training students (ATS), parents, and athletes. School administrators, the school nurse, and even game officials share some of the athletic training program's responsibilities. Duties and responsibilities of each member of the team are interrelated. A school should have a qualified team physician on the sidelines at football games and other high-risk sporting activities. The team physician should be available when any emergency situations arise. Other team physician duties should include supervising pre-participation physicals and medical histories, clearing of players for return to activity after injury, and working with the certified athletic trainer and athletic training students in further development of the athletic training program.

Certified Athletic Trainer

The certified athletic trainer is a highly educated and skilled professional specializing in health care of the physically active. This allied health professional has fulfilled the requirements for national certification, and in some cases, met state licensure requirements. The certification examination consists of a computer-based examination addressing selected content in athletic training curriculum. Within the profession, athletic training practice domains include the following:

- Prevention
- Clinical education and diagnosis
- Immediate care
- Treatment, rehabilitation, and reconditioning
- Organization and administration
- Professional responsibility

Once athletic trainers pass the certification examination, these allied health professionals use the designation certified athletic trainer, or ATC, as their professional credential. Additionally, this credentialed allied health professional needs to confirm that he or she has met state licensure requirements. For specific information, contact the NATA for details regarding state licensure. The ATC is vital to every athletic program. Without an ATC, the coaching staff must assume the responsibilities for the care and prevention of athletic injuries. Research studies have shown that injury rates will increase without an ATC on site at practices and games. The certified athletic trainer serves as the liaison between team physician, coach, parent, athlete, and in some cases, the school administrators. Communications regarding the health of the players must be channeled through the certified athletic trainer in order to have an effective and efficient program. The athletic trainer, especially at the high school level, should maintain contact with parents regarding their child's injury status and ability to return to active competition. Additionally, it may be necessary to notify the appropriate school officials (school nurse, physical education instructor, or principal) of limitations caused by an injury.

During the noncompetitive seasons, the certified athletic trainer should work with the coaches on programs to improve the conditioning level of the team, devising specific programs for certain athletes, assisting athletes recovering from injuries, and monitoring athletes who need to increase their lean body weight or decrease their body fat. Additionally, the certified athletic trainer will assist the coaching staff and the equipment manager on the purchasing and reconditioning of protective equipment. With a letter of delegated authority from the team physician on file, and under his/her direction, the athletic trainer will evaluate and provide first-aid care, initiate an appropriate treatment plan/protocol involving rehabilitative modalities, such as ice, heat, electrical muscle stimulation, ultrasound, design and implement rehab programs based on the physician's protocol, while also applying protective/supportive techniques that will allow the athlete to regain a physically active lifestyle. Additionally duties should include inventory/purchasing of supplies and completing medical/accident record forms and maintaining accurate medical records and documentation.

Other Allied Health Care/Sports Medicine Personnel

- Cardiologist
- Chiropractor
- Dentist
- Emergency medical technician
- Gynecologist
- Internist
- Massage therapists
- Neurosurgeon
- Nurse
- Opthalmologist/optometrist
- Oral surgeon
- Orthopedic surgeon
- Physical therapists/sports therapists
- Podiatrist

Additional Personnel

- Equipment manager
- Exercise physiologist
- Nutritionist
- Sports psychologist
- Strength and conditioning coach/specialist

School Administrators

In the interscholastic and intercollegiate athletic settings, athletic directors, program administrators, or program overseers have the authority and duty to provide a safe working and playing environment. This can be accomplished through strategic planning, defined policies, and clear delineated job responsibilities of all concerned parties.

Athletes

The athlete has the responsibility to maintain good physical condition, practice the techniques taught by the coaches, play by the rules, and follow the instructions of the coaches and the certified athletic trainer.

Parents

Parents can assist in keeping their son or daughter healthy if they are kept updated about the injury or illness. The parents should be provided with information on nutrition and recommended home treatments for injuries. When the involved athlete is a minor, the certified athletic trainer should immediately make the parents aware of the extent of the injury or illness.

Officials

Game officials are responsible for enforcing fair rules, monitoring playing conditions, and cooperating with the certified athletic trainer and physicians when injuries occur and when environmental hazards exist.

Coaches

Coaches have numerous athletic training-related responsibilities. They must plan practices that include conditioning and training of the athlete, and teach techniques and rules of their sport. These practices must be of reasonable duration, taking skill level, fatigue, and environmental conditions into consideration. Coaches are often responsible for selecting, fitting, and maintaining protective equipment. Additionally, the coaching staff must review supervision of practice and game facilities. Coaches must update their education by attending professional development clinics that review rule changes, skill development, first aid/cardiopulmonary resuscitation (CPR) and selected topics in athletic health care. Most importantly, the coach must place the athlete's welfare foremost. The coach must work closely with the team physician and certified athletic trainer in determining what is best for the athlete. Note: If the school does not have a certified athletic trainer, additional duties and responsibilities would then be assumed by the coach.

Athletic Training Student Roles and Responsibilities

The duties of the athletic training student can be defined by his/her interest, experience in allied health care, and desire to gain knowledge of the profession. Once an athletic training student has obtained basic certification from the American Red Cross in first aid and CPR, a supervising certified athletic trainer can assist them in developing skills in the immediate care of injuries, preventive techniques, and basic treatment protocols. Advancement of responsibilities will depend upon the student's ability to master introductory skills in athletic training. Regardless of skill level, athletic training-related techniques should not be attempted without the supervision of an ATC.

Every athletic training student should start by maintaining a professional personal appearance and demeanor. In addition, ensuring a safe and sanitary athletic training area/facility is vital. Because various wounds are treated in the athletic training room, proper cleaning of the facility is critical. One reason is because of the possibility of cross contamination between bodily fluids and the various surfaces in the facility. Other duties assigned to an athletic training student can be inventory control, keeping track of supplies and equipment, and informing the head athletic trainer when inventories are low. The athletic training student should have a checklist of supplies to have on the field or court for games, practices, or road trips. Packing of kits and other preparation activities are good duties for the athletic training student. Additional duties might include preparing a sport/electrolyte drink or water and taking it to the field; making sure there is enough ice, both for treatments and for water coolers; and making sure each athlete has weighed in before and after every practice and documenting weights on the weight charts.

Other than the weight chart documentation, the certified athletic trainer or coach might assign other recordkeeping duties to a capable athletic training student. For example, daily treatments to athletes need to be recorded in a daily log and also in the athlete's medical file. As an athletic training student shows more initiative and competence, he or she may even become involved in taping, wrapping, changing dressings, giving minor treatments, and first-aid procedures. Besides the practical experience gained from working under the supervision of a certified athletic trainer and/or experienced athletic coach, the athletic training student can also benefit from attending educational workshops and reading sport medicine texts and articles.

Athletic Training Facility and Management

Establishing an athletic training room is very important. Athletic training facilities at high schools vary from almost nonexistent to those as modern and spacious as professional/college athletic training rooms. While everyone prefers good working conditions, facilities at some schools will always be less than ideal because of space or budget limitations. However, a resourceful certified athletic trainer will find ways to develop a program regardless of the limited facilities. Typical athletic training rooms include the following areas: administrative office, prevention (taping), hydrotherapy, rehabilitation, treatment (electrical therapy), physician's examination office, and storage room. A review of typical daily tasks for each area is listed below.

Administrative Office
- Document, review, and file all medical records/notes
  1. Physical forms
  2. Injury reports
  3. Treatment forms
  4. Insurance claims
  5. Rehabilitation forms
  6. Physician referral forms
- Maintain a clean organized office and filing system
- Accessibility to phone, fax, and e-mail for business use
- Updated computer, printer, and software

Hydrotherapy Area
- Have whirlpool(s) safety inspected yearly
- Fill whirlpool(s)
  1. Hot: 98/105 degrees
  2. Cold: 55/65 degrees
  3. Ice immersion buckets
- Fill and rotate ice cups
- Make ice bags for treatments
- Clean and disinfect
  1. Whirlpool(s)
  2. Whirlpool benches
  3. Stool(s)

4. Sink and mirror
5. Empty unused ice bags
- Wash and fold towels

Prevention (Taping) Area
- Restock taping areas
- Roll-up elastic/cloth wraps
- Disinfect taping tables
- Prepare heel and lace pads

Rehabilitation Area
- Inspect all equipment
- Make sure all equipment is in its proper place
- Clean and disinfect all equipment

Treatment (Therapeutic Modality) Area
- Have all modalities safety inspected yearly
- Turn off when not in use
- Clean machines
- Wash and fold towels
- Check hydrocollator and paraffin bath levels

Physician's Examination Office
- Confirm specialized medical equipment for physician(s) is available
- Update and restock supplies in physicians medical kit weekly
- Clean surgical trays and refill disinfectants weekly
- Clean, disinfect, restock, and organize exam room after each use

Storage Area
- Keep accurate inventory and notify supervisor when supply is low
- Clean and rotate stock

Additionally, other daily tasks include maintenance of a clean facility, medical record documentation and filing, reviewing supplies and equipment for facility and medical kits, and reviewing new skills and knowledge in the care and prevention of athletic injuries.

Daily Duties
- Disinfect all modalities, equipment, and areas
- Restock athletic training room
- Sweep, mop, empty trash
- Check ice machine/freezer
- Review emergency procedures with staff
- Review/confirm newly acquired skills/knowledge

Supplies and Equipment–Athletic Training Facility
- Adhesive white tape (1", 1.5", 2")
- AED–Automated external defibrillator
- Alcohol pads
- Antiseptic spray
- Athletic training kits
- Adhesive bandages
- Blankets
- Blood pressure cuff/stethoscope
- Biohazard container/bags
- Broom, dustpan, trash can(s)
- CPR mask
- Cervical collar

- Clock
- Crutches, adjustable
- Cups
- Disinfectant spray
- Elastic tape (1", 2", 3")
- Elastic wraps (regular/double length) (2", 3", 4", and 6")
- Eye wash/contact solution
- Face mask cutters
- Gauze pads (sterile and non-sterile) (3" x 3", 4" x 4")
- Hydrocollator cover(s)
- Hydrogen peroxide
- Ice machine and bags
- Latex gloves (sm, med, lg)

- Pen light/otoscope/ophthalmoscope
- Radios (two-way)
- Refrigerator
- Scale
- Scissors (bandage/surgical)
- Soap
- Spine board (head restraints/straps)
- Splints (Sam and vacuum form)
- Tables (treatment, taping, exam)
- Tape cutters
- Thermometer w/covers
- Towels (four dozen)
- Water coolers
- Wheelchair
- Whirlpool(s)

In addition to these items, the athletic training room must adhere to items that are outlined and mandated by the Occupational Safety and Health Administration (OSHA), which are highlighted in Chapter 4. These items deal with the handling of bodily fluids and blood-borne pathogens.

Supplies for Athletic Training Kits

- Athlete's emergency information
- Adhesive white tape (1", 1½", 2")
- Antacid tablets
- Antimicrobial hand wipes/lotion
- Antibacterial/antiseptic cream
- Arm sling/adjustable
- Band-Aids (assorted sizes)
- Bandage scissors/tape cutter
- Biohazard bags
- Blood pressure cuff/stethoscope
- CPR mask
- Cell phone
- Contact lens kit/solution
- Cotton tip applicators
- Elastic wraps (2", 3", 4", 6")
- Electrolyte tablets
- Emergency contact numbers
- Eyewash/sterile saline solution
- Foot powder
- Forms—injury, insurance
- Gauze (sterile/nonsterile pads)
- Heel cups

- Hydrogen peroxide
- Instant cold packs/ice bags
- Latex gloves (sm, med, lg)
- Mirror
- Moleskin
- Mouth shield/protector
- Nail clippers/drill kit
- Paper bag
- Pencil/notepad
- Providine iodine swab sticks/wipes
- Reflex hammer
- Scissors (bandage/surgical)
- Skin lubricant/petroleum jelly
- Sting swabs for insect bites
- Sun lotion
- Tampons
- Tape adherent
- Thermometer
- Tongue depressors
- Tweezers
- Wound closure (Steri-strips)

Athletic Training Room Rules

Once an athletic training room has been established, drafting of rules is very important. First, outline services that will be offered, specific times you will be open, and conduct expected in the athletic training facility. Remember, this is a medical facility, and it should not be used as a gathering place. To prevent misuse, athletic training room rules should be posted and enforced. Some common rules are listed below:

- Coeducational facility
- Treatment provided only to student-athletes
- All medical treatments must be documented by staff
- Athletes should shower after activity before receiving routine treatments
- Athletic training room supplies and equipment will not be removed, except with permission of the certified athletic trainer
- Athletes/sports equipment should be left in the locker room
- Loud music is not permitted
- No swearing or bullying tolerated
- No horseplay
- No pets, unless a certified assistance animal

Rules can be adapted or added, depending on each school's situation.

Recordkeeping

In order to ensure proper treatment of the athlete, careful records should be kept on all athletes. All athletes are required to complete a physical examination and have this medical form on file prior to participation in sporting activities. The team physician may want to keep the original physical examination form in his or her office or in the school nurse's office. However, the certified athletic trainer should have a copy of this medical form and any notations that are significant for the proper care of each athlete. The physical examination form should include past and present condition of the athlete. Additionally, consent to provide treatment and emergency consent forms should be documented and placed in medical records. Any baseline concussion testing that is conducted prior to participation should also be included in the athlete/patient file. Another form that is important in caring for athletic injuries is an accident-injury report form. This form should include these items: athlete's name, sport, date and time of accident/injury, place of injury, mechanism of injury, evaluation of injury, first aid and treatment provided, rehabilitation recommendations, and medical referral to physician. An accident-injury report form is very important, particularly when the injury involves athletic insurance coverage and reporting. Insurance companies require accurate information regarding the reporting of injuries. Check the insurance requirements at your school when designing your school's injury form. The daily treatment form is another important document to be kept when treating injuries. There should be a place on this form for the athlete's name, date and time, treatment provided, protective technique, and rehabilitation procedure utilized. This form should be reviewed often when assessing the progress or lack of progress of an injury. It can tell you which treatment or taping procedure was successful in dealing with that particular injury.

Health Insurance Portability and Accountability Act of 1996 (HIPPA)

The Health Insurance Portability and Accountability Act of 1996 (HIPPA) is a federal regulation was passed to ensure the rights of the athlete (patient) when it comes to health records. Detailed information on HIPAA can be found at www.hipaa.com. This law restricts who has access to the medical records, for a specific length of time, and for what reasons. Typically the athlete signs a waiver to allow physicians and other health care providers to exchange information in order to better serve the injured athlete. This federal law also regulates exactly what information can be exchanged and with whom it can be shared.

Family Educational Right and Privacy Act (FERPA)

FERPA gives parents certain rights with respect to their children's education records. These rights transfer to the student when he or she reaches the age of 18 or attends a school beyond the high school level. Students to whom the rights have transferred are eligible students. (FERPA, 1974).

Legal Issues

Malpractice suits against athletic trainers are on the rise as participation in sports is increasing. Tort is defined as a legal wrong where a remedy will be provided usually in the form of monetary damage (Ray & Konin, 2005). Athletic trainers commit malpractice generally by a tort of negligence.

Negligence

Negligence occurs when an athletic trainer does something a reasonable prudent person wouldn't do or fails to do something a reasonable prudent person would do under these circumstances (Prentice, 2011). The person injured or harmed has to prove that four elements of negligence are fulfilled. The first is a duty of care due because of the connection between the parties. The second step is to show the defendant breached the duty owed to the injured party. Third, proof must be shown that the breach of duty is the reason for harm to the injured party. Fourth, there must be harm, not just potential for harm to have occurred (Osborne, 2001).

The Fundamentals of Athletic Training

Every athlete is entitled to adequate sports-specific conditioning, injury prevention measures, proper treatment of injuries, and a complete rehabilitation experience. Programs for conditioning, injury prevention, therapeutic modalities, and therapeutic rehabilitation are best designed and supervised by highly educated and skilled certified athletic trainers, who have extensive knowledge in first aid, anatomy, physiology, and kinesiology, as well as proper education and training in the use of each of the modalities involved in the treatment/rehab program.

Having a team physician who is well qualified and experienced in sports medicine practices is important. His or her assistance in reducing the risk of injury is vital. In the absence of a physician, the responsibility to give first-aid treatment falls on the certified athletic trainer or coach. The athletic training student should be well qualified and provide assistance when appropriate. Individuals interested in becoming a certified athletic trainer should possess professional skills, knowledge of athletic training, an enjoyment of athletics, an interest in each athlete's well-being, good fitness and personal health, common sense, and a willingness to complete assigned tasks. Avenues of employment for certified athletic trainers include working in educational institutions (secondary and higher education), professional sports associations, sports medicine clinics, hospitals, corporate and industrial settings, the performing arts, and with the military and government agencies,

The certified athletic trainer is a professional who is well educated to carry out the tasks mentioned in the previous sections. A thorough knowledge of anatomy, physiology, physiology of exercise, psychology, first aid, cardiopulmonary resuscitation, nutrition, pharmacology, therapeutic modalities, rehabilitation protocols that include the physical readiness of the returning an injured athlete to activity, and specialized courses in sports medicine are required to carry out these duties. NATA is the administrative organization that dedicates its endeavors to the advancement, encouragement, and improvement of the athletic training profession. A certified athletic trainer who graduates from an accredited athletic training program is eligible to take the certification examination.

Athletic Training Education

Presently, many educational institutions offer athletic training education programs that have met accreditation standards, set forth by the Commission on Accreditation of Athletic Training Education (CAATE). An accredited entry-level education program includes formal instruction in all areas documented in the NATA Athletic Training Educational Competencies. The education program prepares future certified athletic trainers for employment in health care settings. Candidates sitting for the certification examination must graduate from a CAATE-accredited entry-level athletic training education program.

Employment Opportunities: Traditional and Nontraditional

The traditional setting for certified athletic trainers is the college/university site. While this place of employment was the starting point for the profession of athletic training, the job market has expanded and offers a variety of settings for the certified athletic trainer of today. Some fit the traditional model while others are new and not quite as traditional in nature. A list, not comprehensive, of job opportunities is presented.

Secondary Schools

This place of employment is similar to the college/university setting in that the certified athletic trainer works with a school and the sports (team and individual) of that institution. The main difference between the high school setting and the college/university is the size of the staff, with the college/university typically employing more than one certified athletic trainer. While there are high schools that employ more than one certified athletic trainer, the fact is that most high schools in the United States do not employ certified athletic trainers for the health care of their student-athletes. Therefore, this is an excellent place of opportunity for the certified athletic trainer. Also, the certified athletic trainer who is state certified or licensed as a teacher will find school systems more receptive to hiring him or her. Check the particular state laws governing teacher licensure and reciprocity between states.

Professional Sports

This is more traditional in nature, especially with the professional sport teams: football, basketball, baseball, soccer, and hockey. These individuals care for a specific team. On the other hand, some professional sports are geared more toward the individual (i.e., golf, tennis, and track and field). Those certified athletic trainers have the task of providing care to the members of that professional sport and are not typically associated with just one or two individual athletes. Because of the limited number of professional teams and sports, the employment opportunities are restricted compared to other venues with greater numbers.

Sport Medicine Clinics and Hospitals

This is probably the most recognizable nontraditional setting for certified athletic trainers. These sites provide the traditional services offered to athletes, but also can function in the clinic or doctors office as an assistant to other allied health care professionals. Opportunities are varied and state regulations assist in determining the extent of job-related functions. It is best to check with the individual states pertaining to the scope of practice. A typical work day would include time spent in the clinic working with patients and then off-site work with one or more high school athletic programs.

Corporate/Industrial

This is a continuing developing outlet for the certified athletic trainer. The business world has come to realize that a fit and healthy worker is a more productive worker. Also, a variety of exercise opportunities are afforded to the worker. Therefore, injuries occur and the certified athletic trainer is employed to help the worker return to the workforce as quickly as possible. The business world might refer to this as work hardening, corporate health care, etc., but the bottom line is another opportunity for the certified athletic trainer in the nontraditional setting.

Community Recreation Centers

A relatively new site for the certified athletic trainer, but one that is gaining in popularity is the community recreation center. This place of employment would offer the services to a wide range of ages, from the young to the geriatric population. Hours are more uniform and activities would be limited to the extent of the offerings by the particular recreation center.

Other Certifications

Multiple certifications may increase the applicant's chances for a particular job, as long as the employer sees the significance in the credentials and is looking for a person who can do more for the organization. Therefore, an additional credential that a certified athletic trainer should consider would be a certified strength and conditioning specialist. The Colorado-based National Strength and Conditioning Association (NSCA) governs this specialty area. The website for NSCA is www.ncsa.com. NSCA is a nonprofit organization dedicated to unifying its membership and promoting the profession and its principles. Those principles include the relationship to athletic performance, research, and awarding of certifications in the related field of strength training. This certification requires the passage of a written and practical application examination. The exam has multiple-choice questions covering areas such as anatomy, physiology, biomechanics, and nutrition, and a practical application component that tests candidate's knowledge of organization and administration of a strength program, program design, and exercise techniques. With the addition of this certification, the certified athletic trainer can incorporate the knowledge from both athletic training and strength training to design and implement the best rehabilitation program and injury prevention program for their athletes and/or clients.

To succeed as a certified athletic trainer today, one must stay current on the latest techniques in their field. Additionally, the certified athletic trainer who is more diverse and knowledgeable is more valuable to an organization. With these two concepts in mind, the person with a more diverse and unique background will have an edge in the job market. Additionally, multiple certifications should help professionals thrive professionally and be successful in their field. Each certification, including the certified athletic trainer, has continuing education requirements needed to stay abreast of advances in the field and maintain certification status.

Summary

This chapter presented the fundamental concepts of the profession of athletic training and its relationship to the sports medicine team. The necessity for qualified allied health professionals, appropriate supplies, and proper documentation of health care records provides a sound basis for the prevention, care, and treatment of injuries within the active population.

References

American Academy of Orthopedic Surgeons. (2005). *Athletic training and sports medicine.* Chicago: American Academy of Orthopaedic Surgeons.

Anderson, M., & Hall, S. (2005). *Foundations of athletic training.* Baltimore: Lippincott, Williams, & Wilkins.

Board of Certification. (2013). Retrieved from www.bocatc.org/

Family Educational Rights and Privacy Act of 1974. 20 U.S.C. § 1232g; 34 CFR Part 99

Knight, K. (2001). *Assessing clinical proficiencies in athletic training.* Champaign, IL: Human Kinetics.

Mellion, M., Walsh, W., & Shelton, G. (1990) *The team physician's handbook.* Philadelphia: Hanley and Belfus, Inc.

National Athletic Trainers' Association. (March, 2013). Retrieved from http://www.nata.org

National Strength and Conditioning Association. (March 2013). Retrieved from http://www.ncsa.com

Osborne, B. (2001). Principle of Liability for Athletic Trainers: Managing Sport-Related Concussion. *Journal of Athletic Training, 36*(3), 316-321.

Prentice, W. (2006). *Arnheim's principles of athletic training.* St. Louis, MO: McGraw-Hill Higher Education.

Prentice, W. (2011). *Principles of athletic training: A competency-based approach.* New York: McGraw-Hill.

Ray, R. (2005). *Management strategies in athletic training.* Champaign, IL: Human Kinetics.

Taber's Medical Dictionary 22nd Edition. (2012). Philadelphia, PA: F. A. Davis.

Wright, K., Whitehill, W., & Lewis, M. (2005). *Preventive techniques: Taping/trapping techniques and protective devices.* Gardner, KS: Cramer Products.

Review Questions

Completion

1. The athletic training student duties are limited; however, important duties could include _____, _____, and _____ .

2. Just as a coach, the athletic training student should maintain _____certification.

3. Athletic training students can benefit by _____and _____ .

4. A _____ _____ form should be kept to record all treatments given or preventive/supportive techniques applied by the athletic training staff.

5. A _____ is someone who has successfully passed the national certification examination.

Short Answer

1. Coaches play a very important part in the sports medicine program. List two things a coach should know related to the care of an athlete.

2. Name the seven areas of an athletic training facility.

3. List five employment situations where a certified athletic trainer can be employed.

4. List at least five medical personnel who could be members of the sports medicine team.

5. List existing requirements for becoming a certified athletic trainer.

6. What is the mission of NATA?

7. What role do parents play as a member of the sports medicine team?

8. What role do athletes play in health care?

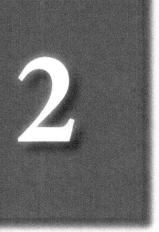

2 Recognition, Evaluation, and Management of Athletic Injuries

Educational Objectives

Upon completing this chapter, the reader will be able to do the following:
- Recognize the signs of life-threatening injuries
- Identify the protocol in first-aid emergency care
- Identify the steps in emergency transportation
- Describe the components of the injury evaluation formats
- Identify types of first-aid splinting equipment
- Describe the basic treatment protocol for athletic injuries

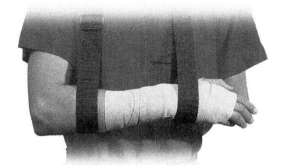

Recognition of Injuries

Primary functions of a certified athletic trainer are to recognize when an injury has occurred, determine the severity of the injury, appropriate referral, and apply proper evaluation/treatment procedures and protocols. The recognition of injuries is a process where the certified athletic trainer, either through direct observation or second hand accounts, determines the probable cause and mechanism of injury. There are two major considerations in emergency evaluations. First, control of life-threatening conditions and activation of emergency medical service, and second, management of non-life-threatening injuries. Referral to a physician is critical when serious injury occurs. If any of the following situations exist, immediate referral is critical (NATA, 2008):
- Loss of respiratory function (breathing)
- Severe bleeding
- Suspicion of intracranial bleeding and/or bleeding from ears, mouth, and/or nose
- Unconsciousness
- Paralysis
- Circulation or neurological impairment
- Shock
- Obvious deformity
- Suspected fracture or dislocation
- Pain, tenderness, or deformity along the vertebral column
- Significant swelling and pain
- Loss of sensation (motor or sensory)
- Loss of motion
- Doubt about the severity of the injury

When a serious injury occurs, the athletic training student should assist qualified health care professionals in providing appropriate care. It is highly encouraged that all medical personnel become familiar with the NATA Emergency Planning in Athletics position statement for specific guidelines (NATA, 2002). The athletic training student's responsibilities in emergency situations include the following:

- Becoming aware of the causes of serious injuries;
- Alerting the certified athletic trainer, athletic coach, and team physician of potential dangers recognizing signs of serious injury
- Implementing a detailed plan to handle emergency transport

First-Aid Emergency Care

Once an injury has occurred, a proper evaluation must be administrated. The American Heart Association (*www.americanheart.org*) and American Red Cross (*www.redcross.org)* have established protocols that will give the athletic trainer the necessary guidance to administer first-aid emergency care. It is critical that certification in American Heart Association BLS for health care providers, cardiopulmonary resuscitation (CPR), automated external defibrillator (AED), and American Red Cross Sport Safety Training (SST) be maintained by certified athletic trainers and athletic coaches. Additionally, a written statement (standing orders and emergency action plan) should be drafted by the team physician that provides direction of how to handle specific injuries. This written document should include the proper protocol for handling life-threatening and non-life-threatening injuries along with protocol to follow in dealing with blood-borne pathogens. This document must be updated and revised frequently in order to stay current with the field.

Emergency Transportation Procedures

There are two points to consider in the area of transportation. The first is the availability of emergency ambulance service and the second is the severity of the injury. The athletic training/sport medicine staff or athletic coaches should never transport an athlete in a private vehicle because of liability issues. With any athletic event or competition, the availability of emergency ambulance service should be present or on call to handle and to transport potential serious injuries. Emergency medical technicians (EMTs) are skilled, practiced professionals who routinely provide advanced medical care and transport injured patients. They have the proper equipment and training to prepare injured athletes for transportation and have vehicles equipped for safe and speedy transport for follow up medical care.

Evaluation of Injuries (Life Threatening and Non-Life Threatening)

Following a written statement (standing orders and emergency action plan) drafted and approved by your team physician and organization, the proper steps in the evaluation of injury can occur. When serious injury is suspected, begin your evaluation with a survey of the scene and then primary survey. Following standard protocols by either the American Heart Association and/or American Red Cross, the primary survey assesses includes the following:

- Airway
- Breathing
- Circulation

To conduct the primary survey, approach the athlete in a calm and reassuring manner. This enhances relaxation and maintenance of the respiratory and circulatory systems. With the primary survey, be prepared to clear and maintain the airway free of potential obstructions such as blood, vomitus, and foreign matter. Assist the patient in finding the most comfortable position for breathing. If necessary, be prepared to provide artificial ventilation or CPR and to activate the emergency medical system.

Once your primary survey is completed and you determine the athlete's condition is non-life threatening, perform a secondary survey. The secondary survey consists of two elements: history and physical examination.

History

The history is that part of the evaluation when the examiner questions the athlete to determine the following:
- Mechanism of injury
- Onset of symptoms
- Location of injury
- Quantity and quality of pain
- Type and location of any abnormal sensations
- Progression of signs and symptoms
- Activities that make the symptoms better or worse
- Nausea
- Weakness
- Dyspnea (shortness of breath)

Physical Examination

The physical examination is your next step. Remember, physical assessment findings may vary tremendously from athlete to athlete, yet still be within a normal range. Factors such as physical activity and exercise may account for this variance. Some signs and symptoms that may vary are respiratory rate, moistness, color and temperature of skin, and pulse rate. Essential to the physical assessment is the evaluation of these vital signs: abnormal nerve response, blood pressure, movement, pulse, respiration, skin color, state of consciousness, and temperature.

Once a life-threatening injury has been ruled out, medical evaluation of non-life-threatening injury must be comprehensive. In the athletic training/sport medicine settings, two formats of evaluation are commonly utilized: HOPS (History, Observation, Palpation, Special Tests) and SOAP Notes (Subjective, Objective, Assessment and Plan).

HOPS Evaluation Format

The first purpose of an evaluation is to determine if a serious injury has occurred. Initially, a fracture should always be suspected. Signs of a fracture include, but are not limited to, direct or indirect pain, deformity, or a grating sound at the injury site. Some fractures are not accompanied by swelling or pain. If a fracture is suspected, the extremity should be splinted and the athlete transported for medical evaluation. Young athletes are especially susceptible to fractures, due to their immature bone structure. Often, ligaments and muscles are stronger than the bones. The evaluation process to help determine the type of injury involves four steps: history, observation, palpation, and special tests.

History

questions asked to determine mechanism of injury

H (History). This involves asking questions of the athlete to help determine the mechanism of injury. Answers to these questions will help the certified athletic trainer in assessing the injury and the physician in a diagnosis:
- Mechanism of injury (How did it happen?)
- Location of pain (Where does it hurt?)

- Sensations experienced (Did you hear a pop or snap?)
- Previous injury (Have you injured this anatomical structure before?)

Observation

checking the involved structure for signs of trauma

O (Observation). The certified athletic trainer should compare the uninvolved to the involved anatomical structure and look for bleeding, deformity, swelling, discoloration, scars, and other signs of trauma.

P (Palpation). Palpation is the physical inspection of an injury. First, palpate the anatomical structures/joints above and below the injured site. Then palpate the affected area. The entire area around the injury may be sore, but the athletic trainer should try to pinpoint the site of severe pain. From knowledge of the human anatomy and injury mechanism, the type and extent of injury can be evaluated. Involve the athlete in the evaluation as much as possible. Using bilateral comparison, these items should be palpated/performed:

Palpation

physical inspection of the injury

- Neurological stability (motor and sensory)
- Circulation function (pulse and capillary refill)
- Anatomical structures (palpate)
- Fracture test (palpation, compression, and distraction)

S (Special tests). With all special tests, the certified athletic trainer is looking for joint instability, disability, and pain. It is possible to further damage an injury through manipulation. Before you attempt to perform the various special tests, make sure you are comfortable and competent in those tests. These tests are well beyond the expertise of an athletic training student. To determine if damage has been done to the anatomical structures, the athletic trainer uses special stress and functional tests to assess disability. These include the following:

Special tests

procedures used to determine joint instability, disability, and pain

- Joint stability (stress applied to determine ligament stability)
- Muscle/tendon (stress applied to determine muscle/tendon stability)
- Accessory anatomical structures (test to determine status of accessory anatomical structures, such as synovial capsule, bursa, menisci, etc.)
- Inflammatory conditions (test to determine if neurological disorders exist and type of inflammation present which can be a significant clue to the type of injury (i.e., intra-articular effusion, extra-articular edema, synovial, etc.)

SOAP Notes Evaluation Format

Assessing an injury using the Subjective, Objective, Assessment, and Plan (SOAP notes) evaluation format is another standardized procedure that provides comprehensive review of probable cause and mechanism of injury. This injury evaluation process is reviewed next.

S (Subjective). Assessment requires the certified athletic trainer to ask detailed questions of pre-existing or existing injuries (history) regarding the following areas:

Subjective

detailed questions designed to gain information

- Previous injury
- How it happened
- When it happened
- What did you feel
- Types of pain
- Where does it hurt
- Sounds/noises

O (Objective). Assessment involves visual, physical, and functional inspections. Items to assess include swelling, deformity, ecchymosis, symmetry, gait/walk, scars, facial expression, circulation, neurological tests (sensation, reflex, motor), bone, soft tissue, range of motion (active, passive, resistive), and sports-specific movements.

A (Assessment). Reviews the probable cause and mechanism of the injury, impressions of injury site (structures involved), severity of injury, and treatment goals.

P (Plan). Should outline appropriate action that should be taken to care for the injury. Initial actions could include: immediate action and referral, modalities utilized, preventive techniques, rehabilitation considerations, and criteria for return to active lifestyle.

Objective

conduct of visual, physical, and functional inspections

Assessment

determines possible cause, severity of injury

Plan

outline of appropropriate action to take

First-Aid Splinting Equipment

A number of different types of equipment are available for the athletic trainer to use in splinting an injured anatomical structure. Splints are intended to protect the injury from further damage. The following is a list of medical splints utilized in emergency situations.

Fixation Splints
These are the most common adaptable splints utilized. Board, wire ladder, structural aluminium malleable splint (SAM), precut cardboard splints, pillow, and blankets are examples of fixation splints. When dealing with suspected upper extremity injuries, the utilization of swathe, sling, and support wrap techniques will aid in extremity immobilization.

Vacuum Splints
These splints are appropriate for dislocations or misaligned fractures and adaptable to any limb angulation.

Pneumatic (Air) Splints
Suited for nondisplaced fractures, air splints are easy to apply. They are no longer the standard of care in athletic injuries.

Traction Splints
Used for long bone fractures (femur and humerus), they prevent fractured bone ends from touching. Advanced medical training is needed to become proficient in application of traction splints.
When using emergency splinting equipment, these key elements should be followed:
- Inspection of the extremity for open wounds, deformity, swelling, and ecchymosis.
- Check pulse, motor, sensation (PMS) and capillary refill of the injured site distal to the injury.
- Cover all wounds with a dry sterile dressing before applying a splint and notify the receiving medical facility of all open wounds.
- Do not move the athlete before splinting extremity injuries unless there is an immediate hazard to the athlete or you.
- Select proper splint in which length and size should cover the immediate injured area, along with all joint structures above and below.
- Place splint beside the injured extremity and then smooth out the contents of the splint. The larger end of splint should be placed proximal to the injury.

- When applying the splint, use your hands to minimize movement. Also, support the injury above and below when applying the splint on the extremity. For stabilization purposes, apply a gentle traction to the limb.
- Secure splint with straps by applying firm compression.
- Again, check pulse, motor, sensation (PMS), and capillary refill at a point distal to the site of injury.
- Apply cold to the injured area and document time. It should be noted that the injury can be X-rayed through some commonly utilized splinting equipment.

Basic Treatment Protocol

Regardless of the mechanism of injury, the athletic training student response to an acute injury should include the basic treatment protocol of protection, rest, ice, compression, elevation, and support (PRICES), followed by referral to a physician. Listed below is a brief description of PRICES protocol.

PRICES

protection, rest, ice, compression, elevation, and support

P–Protection
Once an injury has occurred, protect that injury from further damage by removing the athlete from participation.

R–Rest
After the evaluation is completed, rest the injury. The length of rest is dependent on the severity of the injury; therefore rest could easily be longer than 24 hours.

I–Ice
Apply cold to the injured area. This will aid in controlling bleeding and the associated swelling. This can be performed in one of two ways that are equally effective:
- **Ice packs.** This should be done using plastic bags filled with ice covered with a wet towel. This treatment should be done for 10 minutes, with three hours in between treatment, four times a day.
- **Cold water immersion bath.** This should be done using a bathtub or large basin with a water temperature of between 50 to 60 degrees for 8 minutes, with 3 hours in between treatment, 4 times a day. *Note: Persons with any known circulation problems must avoid ice. If any problems arise, consult a physician.

C–Compression
Utilizing a compression wrap to control swelling, begin the elastic wrap distally (farthest from the heart) to the injury and spiral the wrap toward the heart on the involved extremity. Remove the wrap every three hours. *Note: Compression wraps applied too tight could interfere with circulation or nerve function. Signs and symptoms include extremities turning blue or pink, numbness and tingling of extremities, and increased pain. If the athlete experiences this, remove the elastic wrap and re-evaluation injury!*

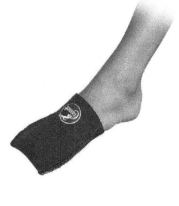

E–Elevation
Keep the injured body part elevated higher than the heart. This will allow gravity to keep excessive blood and associated swelling out of the injured area.

S–Support
Various techniques can be used to support an injury. If necessary, place the injured extremity in a first-aid splint. Examples of other types of support

could include the use of crutches for a lower extremity injury or use of a sling for an upper extremity injury.

Summary

Prior to a sport season, all athletic personnel should be properly trained and certified in the recognition and first-aid procedures of an injured athlete. Following national (CDC, 2013) and specific state guidelines, a detailed plan should be outlined and implemented. The accurate documentation of injury and illness is essential in the process of providing quality health care to the athletic population. Two styles of evaluation formats have been presented in this chapter—HOPS and SOAP notes. There are a number of other formats, but these two provide the most common record documentation format. When treating injuries, the basic treatment protocol of protection, rest, ice, compression, elevation, and support, (PRICES), is a good rule to follow. In all injury management protocols, make sure that you know the proper techniques and work within your knowledge base.

References

Academy of Orthopaedic Surgeons. (2005). *Athletic training and sports medicine.* Chicago, IL: American Academy of Orthopaedic Surgeons.

American Heart Association. (March 2013). *BLS for healthcare providers.* Retrieved from www.heart.org

American Red Cross. (March 2012). *Emergency medical response.* Retrieved from www.redcrosss.org

Anderson, M., & Hall, S. (2012*). Foundations of athletic training.* Baltimore, MD: Lippincott, Williams, & Wilkins.

Centers for Disease Control and Prevention. (March 2103). Retrieved from http://www.cdc.gov

France, R. (2004). *Introduction to sports medicine and athletic training.* New York, NY: Thomson Delmar Learning.

Knight, K. (2010). *Assessing clinical proficiencies in athletic training* (4th ed.). Champaign, IL: Human Kinetics.

National Athletic Trainers Association. (2008). Appropriate Medical Care for the Secondary School-Aged Athlete. *Journal of Athletic Training, 43*(4): 416-427.

National Athletic Trainers' Association. (2002). Position Statement: Emergency Planning in Athletics. *Journal of Athletic Training, 37*(1): 99-104.

National Center for Sport. (March 2012). *PREPARE Sports Safety Courses.* Retrieved from http://www.sportssafety.org

National Conference of State Legislation. (March 2013). *Traumatic brain injury legislation.* Retrieved from www.ncsl.org/issues-research/health/traumatic-brain-injuries

National Safety Council. (2012). *First aid taking action* (2nd ed.). St. Louis, MO: McGraw-Hill Higher Education.

Prentice, W. (2011). *Principles of athletic training: A competency-based approach.* New York: McGraw-Hill.

Ray, R. (2011). *Management strategies in athletic training* (4th ed.). Champaign, IL: Human Kinetics.

Taber's Cyclopedic Medical Dictionary (22nd ed.). (2012). Philadelphia, PA: F. A. Davis.

Williams, J. (1990). *Color atlas of injury in sport.* Chicago, IL: Year Book Medical Publisher, Inc.

Wright, K., Whitehill, W., & Lewis, M. (2005). *Preventive techniques: Taping/wrapping techniques and protective devices.* Gardner, KS: Cramer Products.

Suggested Multimedia Resources

Wright, K., Harrelson, G., Floyd, R., & Fincher, L. (1994). Sports Medicine Evaluation Series (Seven Videos: *The Ankle and Lower Leg; The Knee; The Abdomen; The Thorax; The Shoulder; The Elbow; The Wrist and Hand*). St. Louis, MO: Mosby Year Book, Inc.

Wright, K., & Whitehill, W. (1996). *Sports Medicine Taping Series: Wrapping Techniques for Support & Compression*). St. Louis, MO: McGraw-Hill Higher Education.

Review Questions

Completion

1. When palpating and performing assessment tests, always compare _____ by examining the uninvolved extremity first.

2. Physical inspection begins at the _____ step.

3. List the recommended treatment time for an ice bag: _____.

4. Compression should be accomplished by using an _____ wrap.

Short Answer

1. What is the first step in the injury process?

2. Why are special tests performed?

3. In injury evaluation, what do these terms mean?
    HOPS
    SOAP

4. What are the two major considerations in emergency evaluation?

5. What does the acronym PRICES represent?

6. What are the four different types of splints?

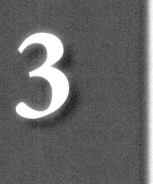

3 Injuries and the Healing Process

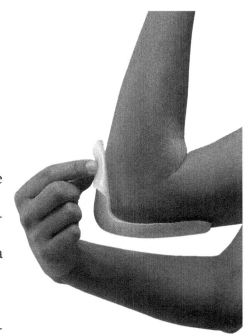

Educational Objectives

Upon completing this chapter, the reader will be able to do the following:
- Describe the inflammation process in the healing of athletic injuries
- Compare obtained values of vital signs to the standard values for a normal patient
- Debate the treatment rationale of ice versus heat application
- Distinguish between acute and chronic injury management
- Explain the principles of physical rehabilitation and range of motion

Successful management of athletic injuries requires an understanding of what happens within the body in response to an injury. An awareness of how healing subsequently occurs is also required. With this, an athletic training student, a coach, or another responder will more fully understand first-aid and follow-up treatments. Treatments can be individually structured to each athlete and to the body part injured. In this chapter, basic principles of healing will be discussed. A complete understanding of this chapter is necessary before advancing to further chapters.

Healing

the process by which the body repairs damaged tissue

The Inflammation Process

When an athletic injury occurs, whether it is a strain, sprain, contusion, or open wound, the body immediately begins a process that eventually results in healing. This process is known as inflammation. While many people feel that inflammation is a negative aspect of injury, it is absolutely essential for complete healing of an injured anatomical structure. In an acute injury, such as a muscle strain or ligament sprain, tissue is torn, capillaries are damaged, and cells die because of the interference in the blood and oxygen supply.

In response, the body reacts by sending specialized cells into the injury area in an attempt to limit damage and to begin healing. Among the functions of these cells is the initiation of blood clotting. In an attempt to limit the size of the damaged area, the body also reacts by contracting muscles in the injured area. This involuntary muscle spasm splints the area to restrict further movement and also reduces the local blood flow.

Inflammation

one component of the healing process, where the body begins to repair itself

In acute injuries, the trauma and the body's reaction to the trauma, result in the five cardinal signs of inflammation: pain, swelling, redness, heat, and loss of function. The pain is caused by increased pressure on nerve endings from internal hemorrhage and from the cellular response to lack of oxygen.

Three phases of the healing process

- inflammation
- tissue repair
- regeneration

Swelling, or edema, is caused by the accumulation of fluids in the damaged area. Hemorrhage, lymph fluid, and synovial fluid contribute to the swelling, increasing pressure on nerve endings. Gravity could also increase swelling if the limb is not elevated. Redness and a feeling of heat (warmth) occur once the healing process begins. The redness is due to the increased blood supply as the body attempts to provide the injury site with nutrients for repair. Loss of function will result in the athlete's inability to utilize the injured anatomical structure.

When referring to an athletic injury, biological removal of unwanted items from the injured area precedes rebuilding. All the fluids and dead cells that have resulted in swelling must be removed from the injury site by the circulatory and lymphatic systems before oxygen and nutrient-supplying capillaries can be formed to assist repair. Removing the waste products and allowing oxygen and other nutrients to get to the damaged area will create an ideal environment for the formation of replacement tissue. Scar tissue is usually the end result due to ideal situations for regeneration not often being present.

Vital Signs

When evaluating an injured athlete, it is essential that one has a sound understanding of how to check the athlete's vital signs and the standard values for the vital signs. By knowing what the standard values are, it is easier to distinguish whether an athlete's vital signs are abnormal. Vital signs would be evaluated in the primary survey of an emergency evaluation and, if necessary, are monitored throughout the entire evaluation and the initial treatment.

Vital signs

those measures that monitor life, such as heart rate, breathing, pulse

Pulse
Adult 60-80 beats per minute, Child 80-100 beats per minute

Rapid but weak pulse could indicate shock, bleeding, diabetic coma, and/or heat exhaustion. A rapid and strong pulse typically indicates heat stroke and/or severe fright. A strong but slow pulse usually indicates a skull fracture and/or stroke. No pulse indicates cardiac arrest and/or death. The two most convenient sites for taking the pulse are the neck (carotid artery) and the wrist (radial artery).

Respiration
Adult 12-20 breaths per minute, Child 20-25 breaths per minute

Breathing that is shallow usually indicates shock. Irregular or gasping breath could be cardiac related. Frothy blood from the mouth typically indicates a chest fracture (rib fracture) in the upper lateral portion of the chest (arm pit). Measurement for respiration is taken by watching, feeling and counting the rise and fall of the chest.

Temperature
(Degrees Fahrenheit) Oral 98.6, Rectal 99.6, Axillary 97.6

Hot, dry skin usually indicates disease, infection, and/or overexposure to environmental heat. Typically, cool, clammy skin is an indicator of trauma, shock, and/or heat exhaustion. Overexposure to cold is displayed by cool, dry skin.

Skin Color
Red skin indicates heat stroke, diabetic coma, and/or high blood pressure. White (pale) skin means that the individual has insufficient circulation, shock, fright, hemorrhage, heat exhaustion, and/or insu-

lin shock. Blue (cyanotic) skin indicates circulated blood is poorly oxygenated. The non-white athlete will still exhibit a paling of the skin, but you should examine the inner lip, gum area and fingernail beds.

Pupils
Constricted (sunlight), Dilated (dark room), or Unequal
In traumatic situations, pupils that are constricted usually indicate injury to the central nervous system and/or intake of a depressant drug. Dilated pupils (one or both eyes) could indicate head injury, shock, heat stroke, hemorrhage, and/or intake of a stimulant drug. When pupils fail to accommodate to light or are unequal this could indicate brain injury, intake of alcohol, or drug poisoning. PEARL is also an accepted protocol in the examination of the eyes. This stands for pupils equal and reactive to light.

State of Consciousness
When evaluating an individual's level of consciousness (LOC), three items to review are the athlete's mental awareness, memory and ability to recall, and response to commands, such as direction, events, etc. This can also be grouped under the initials AVPU—alert, verbal, responds to pain, and unresponsive.

Movement
Movement is classified into four basic patterns: active (athlete provides movement), passive (athletic trainer moves the body part), assistive (athlete trainer assists the athlete with movement), and resistive (athletic trainer provides resistance to oppose the movement of the body part).

Abnormal Nerve Stimulation
When evaluating nerve stimulation, always check for motor (movement) and sensory (feeling) to determine if the affected area has nerve damage. Ensuring that the athlete is able to contract the affected muscle confirms this. To check sensation, touch the affected body part and ask the athlete to distinguish the quality of sensation (i.e., sharp vs. dull).

Blood Pressure
When the heart contracts, systolic pressure can be determined; as the heart relaxes, diastolic pressure can be determined. Normal blood pressure in healthy adults is usually 120/80 mmHg (systolic/diastolic).

Treatment Rationale: Ice vs. Heat

When treating athletic injuries, selection of ice or heat application as a modality is critical. In most situations, ice should be used for the first 48 to 72 hours. Then, re-evaluate the injury and determine if it is still increasing in size (due to swelling) or is warm to the touch. If either condition exists, continue the use of ice. The philosophy of the medical staff will indicate when to use ice or heat. Listed below is a brief outline of types of ice and heat applications.

Application of ICE
The basic physiological changes that occur through the use of ice on an injury include the following:
- Reduced pain at the injury site
- Reduced tissue's metabolic need for oxygen
- Reduced blood flow to the injury site

Cold Packs

There are a variety of different types of cold packs on the market, including chemical ice bags that can be refrozen in a freezer, and traditional ice bags, which are crushed ice placed into a plastic bag. Either can be used for initial first-aid or follow-up treatments, but research has shown that the traditional ice bag is safer for the patient with less chance of causing frostbite.

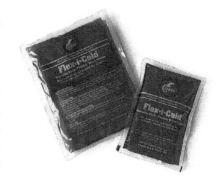

Ice Bags

The best option for acute application of ice. This should be done using plastic bags filled with ice (ideally crushed ice instead of cubed ice) covered with a wet towel. This treatment should be done for 10 minutes, with three hours in between treatment, four times a day. Of importance to note is that any persons with known circulation or sensation problems must avoid ice altogether, regardless of the specific type of ice application. In addition, athletes should not fall asleep while being treated with an ice bag.

Chemical Ice Packs

This is the most economical application of ice. Because of the danger of frostbite, the ice pack should not be applied directly to the skin. Also, the cold pack should be placed on the injury, not under the body where pressure can magnify possible damaging effects such as blistering or burning. Over a period of time, reusable cold packs may be more convenient than ice. Instant cold packs are also available for times when prefrozen packs are not practical, but these are expensive, and chemical burns can result if a leak occurs in the container.

Ice Massage

The technique of rubbing ice over an injured area is called ice massage. Applied by the athlete when possible, this treatment is applied directly to the skin. A paper or insulated cup is filled with water, then frozen. The cup is gradually peeled back as the athlete massages the injury site and the ice melts. The treatment should last from 5-10 minutes depending on the depth and severity of the injury. To prevent skin damage the athlete should move the ice cup continuously with a circular or back-and-forth motion. Ice massage should be avoided over bony areas.

Cryotherapy

cold therapy

Cold Whirlpool/Cold Water Immersion

Before immersing the injured extremity in cool water, the water temperature in a whirlpool tank or bucket should be 50-60 degrees Fahrenheit. Under supervised conditions, the injured extremity is kept in the cool water for five to fifteen minutes. In certain situations, a thermal barrier (e.g., toe cap) is placed around the extremity for patient comfort. With physician approval, the injured athlete then performs rehabilitation movements. The whirlpool offers a massaging effect.

Cold Spray

In certain situations, the use of cold sprays (ethyl chloride) can be beneficial to reduce pain but has little effect on swelling. Using caution, apply the spray to the affected area for no longer than 10 seconds. Since damage to the skin can occur, read the instructions prior to application. Because this technique only cools the surface, it is not nearly as effective as cold treatments. In certain supervised situations, this application of ice is utilized in spray and stretch techniques.

Application of HEAT

Heat should not be used in the first 48-72 hours or longer, unless advised by a physician or certified athletic trainer, due to the increase in swelling and resultant healing time of the tissues. The basic physiological changes that occur through the use of heat on an injury includes the following:

- Increased blood flow to the injured area
- Reduced muscle stiffness
- Muscular relaxation

Hot Packs

Pre-heated commercial hot packs are an efficient way to apply moist heat. Towels are used to insulate the pack and protect the skin from burning. Towels soaked in very hot water have the same effect as hot packs during the period of follow-up treatments, provided that proper insulation is placed between the skin and the heat. It should be noted that the heat penetration of hot packs is limited and is not a substitute for proper warm up and stretching.

Hot Whirlpool

Also used for cold water immersion, the whirlpool bath is a popular method for warm water immersion. Used as a follow-up treatment, the disadvantages of whirlpool treatment include placing the injured part in a nonelevated, dependent position. Also, the equipment must be thoroughly cleaned daily to prevent the spread of disease. Duration of the treatment and temperature depend on the area of the body to be treated. Buckets of warm water can provide the same water-immersion effect as whirlpools. However, the whirlpool also offers a massaging effect.

Application of ICE and HEAT

Contrast bath. The contrast bath is a follow-up treatment that combines hot and cold water immersion. In a nongravity-dependent position, the use of moist heat pack and cold/ice packs are commonly utilized. While this is a traditional treatment approach that has seen positive results, research does not support it's use for the goal of removing swelling. It appears that the traditional thought of a vascular "pumping" action due to the alternating vasodilation and vasoconstriction of blood vessels does not occur to a degree high enough to cause changes in the amount of inflammation in a joint.

Additional Therapeutic Techniques

Exercise

Too often, exercise is overlooked as a treatment. The movement of the body by the muscles increases circulation at a deeper level than the modalities that have been discussed. Exercise is used to maintain or increase strength and to regain lost range of motion in order to assist in the healing process.

Therapeutic Modalities

Various electrical modalities are used to decrease pain, swelling, and muscle spasm. Therapeutic modalities may be utilized as adjuncts to therapeutic exercise by decreasing pain and swelling and by enhancing range of motion, strength and flexibility. Modalities may consist of heat, cold, light, air, water, massage and electricity. When determining which modalities to use, target the tissue to be treated, determine desired treatment effect, and again, look for indications and contraindications. Below is a brief list of some commonly utilized modalities:

- Ultrasound
- Electrical stimulating currents
- Shortwave and microwave diathermy
- Ultraviolet therapy
- Low-power lasers

Massage

Because the friction of massage increases the temperature of the tissues and, therefore, increases local circulation, massage can be considered as a heat treatment. Massage is used as a follow-up treatment for musculoskeletal injuries and for scar tissue/adhesion breakdown. Besides increasing temperature, a massage can help to relax a muscle spasm in injured muscles. As with other heat treatments, massage started too soon after an injury can restart internal bleeding. Additionally, massage is often used as an adjunct to stretching and warm-up exercises in many sports and can assist the body in the removal of toxins from an injured site.

Counterirritants

Counterirritants are substances that when applied to the skin cause a reaction. This reaction can produce a sensation that is stronger than the sensation of minor pain. Long used by athletes, analgesic balms irritate the skin to provide a perception of warmth, which can help relax tight, aching muscles. Penetration of these analgesics is minimal. Their advantages include ease of application and availability. Some counterirritants can also provide a cooling sensation. Care should be taken not to apply counterirritants to an open wound.

Joint Mobilization

This technique is used to improve joint mobility by restoring accessory movement to allow non-restricted, pain-free range of motion. Under the direction of a highly qualified and trained allied health professional, joint mobilization is an effective therapeutic treatment.

Acute vs. Chronic Injury Management

Acute Injuries

Regardless of the mechanism of injury, the response to an acute injury should include the basic treatment of protection, rest, ice, compression, elevation, and support (PRICES), followed by referral to a physician or certified athletic trainer. Listed below is a brief description of the PRICES protocol.

Acute

quick onset,
short duration

Protection. Once an injury has occurred, protect that injury from further damage by removing the athlete from participation.

Rest. After the evaluation is completed, rest the injury. The length of rest is dependent on the severity of the injury, therefore rest could easily be longer than 24 hours.

Ice. Apply cold to the injured area. This will aid in controlling bleeding and the associated swelling. Apply in one of two ways:

Compression. Utilizing a compression wrap to control swelling, begin the elastic wrap distally (farthest from the heart) to the injury and spiral the wrap toward the heart. Remove the wrap every 4 hours. *Note: Compression wraps applied too tight could interfere with circulation or nerve function. Signs and symptoms include extremities turning blue or pink, numbness and tingling of extremities, and increased pain.*

Elevation. Keep the injured body part elevated higher than the heart. This will allow gravity to keep excessive blood and associated swelling out of the injured area.

Support. Various techniques can be used to support an injury. If necessary, place the injured athlete on crutches for a lower extremity injury or use of a sling for an upper extremity injury. This external support will allow the injury to be managed with better control.

Chronic Injuries

The management of chronic injuries is characterized by the continued use of PRICES, but is coupled with exercise, therapeutic modalities, heat, and contrast bath treatments. Even though these injuries can be challenging, the athlete's return to physical activity without chronic pain and disability if important.

Physical Rehabilitation

The goal of a sound physical rehabilitation program is to return the injured athlete to pre-injury levels of strength, power, endurance, flexibility, and confidence as quickly and safely as possible. A rehabilitation program focuses on the injured body part and also with preventing de-conditioning of the rest of the body. If the athlete returns to activity without undergoing physical rehabilitation, the athlete could easily become reinjured. Typically, the injured athlete is an exceptional patient, motivated to get well and to overcome the injury. Some athletes will need encouragement daily during their rehabilitation, while others will need to be restrained from trying to rush their recovery. Open communication between the coach and the sports medicine team members regarding the athlete's progress is critical.

In an ideal situation, a certified athletic trainer will arrange an individual rehabilitation program based upon the physician's protocol standards. With an approved rehabilitation program, the two principles that must be observed are that pain should be avoided, and the athlete must be encouraged to follow the program. However, an aggressive rehabilitation program will require a particular exercise program by the athlete at a level slightly less than what causes pain. Daily adherence to a rehabilitation program benefits the athlete in several ways. First, the athlete stays in the habit of working out. Also, daily exercise will result in tangible results; missing even one day can affect strength or conditioning. Psychologically, the athlete will feel better about himself/herself if allowed to participate in his/her own recovery, rather than watching practice. The athletic trainer should set specific times each day for the athlete to work on the rehabilitation program. A comprehensive rehabilitation program is critical to the injured athlete. In designing this program, the following five phases of physical rehabilitation need to be addressed:

Chronic
of longer duration, repeating

- Post-surgical/acute injury
- Early exercise
- Intermediate exercise
- Advanced exercise
- Initial sports re-entry

An athlete will move through all five phases of the rehabilitation program on the way to complete recovery. Everyone, including the athlete, must keep in mind that each athlete and each injury is different. Various rates of recovery should be expected.

While rehabilitation uses prescribed exercise to return individuals to activity, rehabilitation techniques can also help prevent injuries. In planning a physical rehabilitation program, the athletic trainer must deal with decreasing pain, effusion, and the inflammatory response to trauma. Once this is addressed, returning the athlete to a pain-free, active range of motion that will increase muscular strength, power, and endurance to the injured anatomical structures is critical. The three basic components of any physical rehabilitation program are listed here:

- Therapeutic exercise
- Therapeutic modalities

- Athlete education

When determining the purpose of an exercise, always consider joint range of motion, muscle flexibility, muscular strength, power and endurance, balance, proprioception, and kinesthetic awareness and cardiovascular fitness (total body conditioning). Progressive resistive exercises are used to increase muscular strength, power, and endurance. Finally, it must be understood that functional and sport specific rehabilitation programs need to be incorporated to insure that the athlete can perform the functions that are required in their particular sport.

Range of Motion

Assessing joint range of motion (ROM) is critical in evaluating injuries. The athletic trainer should gain experience in using a goniometer, an instrument that objectively measures joint range of motion. Typical ranges of motion for anatomical joints are listed below:

Range of motion

the normal movement of a joint

Ankle
Dorsiflexion–20 degrees
Plantarflexion–45 degrees
Inversion–40 degrees
Eversion–20 degrees

Knee
Flexion–140 degrees
Extension–0 degree

Hip
Flexion–125 degrees
Extension–10 degrees
Adduction–40 degrees
Abduction–45 degarees

Shoulder
Flexion–180 degrees
Extension–45 degrees
Adduction–40 degrees
Abduction–180 degrees
Internal rotation–90 degrees
External rotation–90 degrees

Elbow
Flexion–140 degrees
Extension–0 degrees

Forearm
Pronation–80 degrees
Supination–85 degrees

Wrist
Flexion–80 degrees
Extension–70 degrees
Adduction–45 degrees
Abduction–20 degrees

General Musculoskeletal Disorders

When treating injuries, an understanding of specific disorders is important. Review these disorders and discuss the specific treatment required with your certified athletic trainer and team physician.
- **Arthritis:** inflammation of a joint
- **Atrophy:** decreasing in size of a developed organ or tissue due to degeneration of cells
- **Bursitis:** inflammation of a bursa sac

- **Contracture:** fibrosis of muscle tissue producing shrinkage and shortening of the muscle without generating any strength
- **Contusion:** a bruise; an injury usually caused by a blow in which the skin is not broken
- **Dislocation:** displacement of one or more bones or a joint, or of any organ from the original position
- **Epicondylitis:** inflammation of the epicondyle and the tissues adjoining the epicondyle to the humerus (pitcher's elbow-medial epicondyle, tennis elbow-lateral epicondyle)
- **Fascitis:** inflammation of a fascia
- **Myositis:** inflammation of muscle tissue
- **Myositis ossificans:** inflammation of muscle, with formation of bone
- **Sprain:** a stretching or tearing of joint structures (ligaments and joint capsules)
- **Strain:** a stretching or tearing of muscles and tendons
- **Subluxation:** a partial or incomplete dislocation
- **Synovitis:** inflammation of the synovial membrane
- **Tendinitis:** inflammation of the tendon
- **Tenosynovitis:** inflammation of tendon sheath

Summary

The healing process begins almost immediately after the injury occurs. Athletic trainers must recognize the components of that process and provide the best environment and care. Vital signs help assess the athlete's condition. This chapter also identified the application of both heat (thermotherapy) and cold (cryotherapy) for either acute or chronic injuries. Finally, with most injuries, rehabilitation is a vital component of the healing process. Rehabilitation is more successful when both exercise and modality are combined. With all rehabilitation, the athletic trainer should work closely with the physician and physical therapist.

References

Anderson, M., Parr, G., & Hall, S. (2009). *Foundations of athletic training: Prevention assessment, and management* (4th ed.). Philadelphia, PA: Williams & Wilkins.

Barker, S., Wright, K., & Wright, V. (2001). *Sports injuries 3D* (3rd ed.). Gardner, KS: Cramer Products, Inc.

Knight, K., & Draper, D. (2008). *Therapeutic modalities: The art and science.* Baltimore, MD: Lippincott Williams & Wilkins.

Magee, D. (2002). *Orthopedic physical assessment* (4th ed.). Philadelphia, PA: W.B. Sanders.

Pfieffer, R., & Mangus, B. (2011). *Concepts of athletic training* (6th ed.). Boston, MD: Jones and Bartlett.

Prentice, W. (2011). *Arnheim's principles of athletics: A competency-based approach* (14th ed.). St. Louis, MO: McGraw-Hill Higher Education.

Prentice, W. (2011). *Rehabilitation techniques in sports medicine* (5th ed.). St. Louis, MO: McGraw-Hill Higher Education.

Prentice, W. (2009). *Therapeutic modalities: For sports medicine and athletic training* (6th ed.). St. Louis, MO: McGraw-Hill Higher Education.

Starkey, C., Brown, S., & Ryan, J. (2010). *Examination of orthopedic and athletic injuries* (3rd ed.). Philadelphia, PA: F. A. Davis.

Stedman's medical dictionary for the health professions and nursing (7th ed.). (2011). Baltimore, MD: Williams & Wilkins.

Wright K., Whitehill W., & Lewis, M. (2003). *Preventive techniques: Taping/wrapping techniques and protective devices.* Gardner, KS: Cramer Products.

Review Questions

Completion

1. The body's reactions to trauma are ____, ____, ____, ____, and ____.

2. Redness and a feeling of warmth around an injury are signs of an increase of ____ to that body part.

3. Normal pulse readings for adults are _____ and children are _____.

4. Normal blood pressure of a healthy adult is ___/___.

5. Ice is used initially on an injury to reduce _____, _____, and ____.

6. Range of motion of a joint can be measured by using a _____.

7. All the fluids and dead cells that have resulted in swelling must be removed from the injury site by the _____ and _____ systems.

8. A rehabilitation program should not only focus on the injured body part, but also on preventing _____ of the rest of the body.

Short Answer

1. What five phases of physical rehabilitation need to be included in a comprehensive rehabilitation program?

2. List three physiological changes associated with ice.

3. List three physiological changes associated with heat.

4. Explain the difference between arthritis and bursitis.

4 Biohazardous Protocols and Skin Conditions

Educational Objectives

Upon completing this chapter, the reader will be able to do the following:
- Recognize the need to comply with Occupational Safety and Health Administration (OSHA) guidelines
- Demonstrate preventive and protective measures in waste management
- Identify blood-borne pathogens commonly observed in athletic training
- Recognize the National High School Federation and National Collegiate Athletic Association rules as they relate to biohazardous materials
- Recognize the classification and management of wounds
- Identify the various skin conditions that are common in athletic training situations

Occupational Safety and Health Administration

Standard Precautions and Transmission-based Precautions—Guidelines Established for the Prevention of the Spread of Infectious Materials.

Although Occupational Safety and Health Administration (OSHA) regulations concerning exposure to blood-borne pathogens (BBP) in the workplace were established in 1992, confusion and myths still exist. Many schools and companies do not understand the regulations and are not in compliance. The fact that a school or company does not fully understand the standard will not protect it from enforcement penalties should OSHA investigate adherence/compliance with regulations. Risk of actual infection with a blood-borne disease is still minimal, but is growing, especially from Hepatitis B; currently there are nearly 38,000 new cases diagnosed each year. Hepatitis B is a viral infection that affects the liver and can be fatal. Hepatitis B can be prevented through a series of 3-4 vaccinations given over a 6-month period. Hepatitis B vaccination is required in most state for health care workers and is also required for students by many public schools and universities. The Centers for Disease Control and Prevention (CDC) estimates that exposure to Hepatitis B is 100 times more likely than exposure to HIV/Aids. Also, it is estimated by the CDC in 2013 that over 1 million people in the United States are living with human immunodeficiency virus (HIV), including more than 200,000 (18%) who are unaware of their infection. It is estimated that there are upwards of 40,000 new cases each year. Currently, there is no cure or vaccine for this deadly disease. How many new cases of HIV develop each year is unknown, but the total number of known cases has increased. While the OSHA regulations are time consuming to follow, they aim to be effective in reducing the risk of infection even further and, therefore, will help stop the

> **Universal precautions**
>
> guidelines established for the prevention of the spread of infectious disease

spread of blood-borne diseases. Some frequently asked questions regarding OSHA standards include the following:

What are the OSHA blood-borne pathogens standards? OSHA Regulation 1910.1030, Occupational Exposure to Blood-borne Pathogens, sets forth required procedures for protecting employees of any type of company, organization, or institution against accidental exposure to blood-borne pathogens. This standard was first published in the *Federal Register* on December 6, 1991 and became effective March 6, 1992. For access to current blood-borne pathogens standards, contact your local health department or access the CDC website at www.cdc.gov.

Is my school covered by this standard? If your school has employees who, in the course of the work, can reasonably be expected to come into contact with human blood, certain body fluids, or infectious waste, the school must comply with the provisions of OSHA 1910.1030.

In a scholastic setting, who might be at risk of exposure? The most obvious employees are certified athletic trainers, coaches, and school nurses who are first responders to athletic or other injuries. The basketball or wrestling coach dealing with a bloody nose or split lip is considered to be in the presence of infectious material. The athletic trainer treating a common abrasion makes his or her employer subject to the standard. Less obvious are teachers providing first aid, the custodial personnel required to mop the gym floor or wrestling mat upon which blood has been spilled, and the laundry workers who must handle blood soaked uniforms. All of these employees are covered by the standard, and provided its protection.

Contamination
the process of infection

Are game officials and referees considered employees? Yes. As soon as a high school hires them to work a game or match, they are technically considered to be employees of the school and the protections spelled out in the standard must be provided to them.

What are the basic provisions of OSHA 1910.1030? The blood-borne pathogens standard involves seven very precisely defined areas discussed below:
- Scope (identifies employees covered)
- Exposure control plan (a written, site-specific plan outlining the steps to be taken to minimize employee exposure to blood-borne pathogens)
- Methods of compliance (written procedures on how to control exposure)
- Vaccinations and medical evaluations (outlines Hepatitis B vaccination requirements and post exposure medical evaluation and follow-up)
- Information and training (explains requirements for communicating standard to employees)
- Record keeping (defines records that must be kept)
- Dates (provides schedule of implementation)

Can the NCAA, NAIA, National Federation or any other national sport governing body issue rules, which supersede the OSHA standard? All have issued guidelines covering exposure to infectious substances. In general, these are designed to protect student athletes and do not address the total requirements of protecting employees. No guidelines supersede the OSHA standard, unless those guidelines are more stringent than OSHA policy.

If my school is in compliance with regulations of its national governing body, is it in compliance with the OSHA Standard? No. Unless the regulations of the organization are at least as comprehensive as OSHA 1910.1030 they would not be a substitute for them.

Can our team's athletic trainer, manager or coach remove blood from a player's uniform and be in compliance with the OSHA Standard? There is nothing in the standard, which specifically prohibits the removal of blood from uniforms. However, the standard does stipulate the only approved method of removing blood from a uniform is to put the uniform through a complete wash cycle with a commercial laundry detergent. Even though participants and other associated individuals could conceivably be exposed through an improperly disinfected uniform, OSHA would most likely discourage the practice of removing blood from uniforms with a chemical spot remover.

What about spraying a disinfectant on the blood spot? This method is not approved as an effective means to disinfect a potentially contaminated uniform. Blood on uniforms is absorbed by thousands of threads made of microscopic fibers. The extent to which a disinfectant will kill viruses and tuberculosis bacilli has not been verified. Presently utilized CDC testing methods apply to hard, non-absorbent surfaces only.

Blood-Borne Pathogens

As certified athletic trainers, our primary concern is the health of our athletes. However, we must also be concerned for our own personal safety. In 1992, OSHA issued regulations regarding health care workers and the handling of blood-borne pathogens. The blood-borne pathogens of most concern are Hepatitis B and Hepatitis C, which are much easier to transfer than another blood-borne pathogen, the HIV virus, which is not easily transferred in the athletic setting. These are of special concern to the certified athletic trainer since it is common for the certified athletic trainer to come in contact with blood and other body fluids on a daily basis. It is possible the very athletes we are trying to help may infect us and this contamination is potentially lethal. Consistent with universal precautions, the certified athletic trainer should always know and practice proper preventive measures. Fortunately, OSHA has provided basic guidelines for the health care professional. Latex gloves provide a suitable barrier for athletic trainers, but occasionally a person is allergic to latex or NRL (natural rubber latex). Those allergic reactions might be as mild as an itching sensation, to redness and swelling of the affected parts, to the more severe symptoms of impaired breathing and the need for advanced medical care. For more information on latex allergy go to the website www.osha.gov/STLC/latexallergy.

Transmission of disease

methods by which disease can be transferred from one individual to another

Preventive and Protective Measures in Waste Management

A certified athletic trainer can be exposed to blood-borne pathogens in a variety of ways. The most obvious is treating an athlete with some sort of bloody wound. Other situations would include serum fluid in blisters and vomitus with an ill athlete. Only if saliva were to have a bloody component would it also be included in fluids to be cautious in handling. Given these exposure opportunities, the athletic trainer should take proper precautions. First, wear latex or hypoallergenic gloves when working on athletes with exposed body fluids. The use of gloves provides a barrier between you and the wound or bodily fluid you are treating. Gloves should be worn at all times when evaluating an athlete, especially when the possibility of an undiscovered, open wound may exist. When wearing protective gloves, there are some general guidelines an athletic trainer should follow. The protective value of the gloves diminishes after 10-15 minutes of wearing them. If gloves should tear, replace them immediately. When choosing gloves, a certified athletic trainer should select a size that fits his or her hands. After use, the gloves and all contaminated materials should be disposed of properly in a biohazard infectious waste container. The next step the athletic trainers should follow is cleaning of the contaminated athletic training room. An effective preparation is one part bleach to 10 parts water

Blood-borne pathogens

those microorganisms that are carried in the blood throughout the body solution. In addition to the bleach solution, you can buy commercially prepared products that have the same effects. To prepare the solution, add 1 ounce of bleach to 10 ounces of water in a spray bottle. The bleach should be mixed with cool water. Warm or hot water deactivates the bleach's basic cleaning agent, hypochlorite. Label the bottle and store it so it is accessible only to those who are going to use it. This solution mixture is good only one day, so it should be made daily. In using the bleach/water solution to clean up body fluids, the following procedure is recommended:

Standard precautions

guidelines established for the prevention of the spread of infectious materials

- Put on protective gloves.
- Absorb fluids with paper towels.
- Saturate the area with bleach solution and allow soaking before absorbing it with another paper towel.
- Scrub the area with bleach solution and then soap and water, using a paper towel.
- Rinse the area.
- All soiled materials, including gloves, should be placed in the biohazard bag/container.
- Wash hands thoroughly after disposal of materials.

National High School Federation Rules

In 1994, the National Federation of State High School Associations (NFSHSA) www.NFHS.org, adopted its nine-point communicable disease procedures. This document outlines the protocols that should be followed in the handling of bodily fluids. The nine points include the following:
- Stop bleeding and remove blood from uniforms.
- Use precautions when handling bodily fluids.
- Wash body surfaces exposed to bodily fluids.
- Clean all surfaces and equipment before resuming play.
- Rinse the area thoroughly.
- Use artificial ventilation devices when performing CPR.
- All soiled materials, including gloves, should be placed in a biohazard bag/container.
- Properly clean and/or dispose of blood-soaked towels.
- Follow accepted guidelines for controlling bleeding.

These guidelines are not identical to the OSHA guidelines and are not universal precautions. The safety of all people involved is the most important point to remember. Therefore, follow guidelines that provide protection and safety to participants and associated personnel. In addition to establishing communicable disease procedures, the NFSHSA also has established specific rules on players who are bleeding. For more information, contact the NFSHSA regarding the specifics of each sport.

Classification and Management of Wounds

Wounds involve a compromise to the integument (skin) system. Once the skin is penetrated, various types of wounds could exist. Listed below is a classification of the five types of wounds.
- Abrasions
- Avulsions
- Incisions
- Lacerations
- Punctures

Once an individual has suffered a wound, immediate treatment should be taken and appropriate steps to eliminate infection incorporated. A properly stocked and readily accessible wound management kit is the first step in the treatment of any type of wound. This kit should include the following:

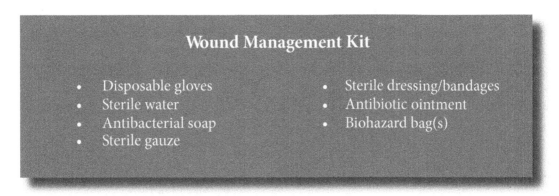

Wound Management Kit

- Disposable gloves
- Sterile water
- Antibacterial soap
- Sterile gauze
- Sterile dressing/bandages
- Antibiotic ointment
- Biohazard bag(s)

Remember, when treating any type of wound, always wear protective gloves, follow current OSHA guidelines and refer the athlete(s) for medical evaluation.

Also, observe the wounds daily for any of the following signs of infection:

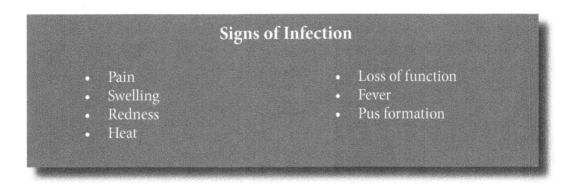

Signs of Infection

- Pain
- Swelling
- Redness
- Heat
- Loss of function
- Fever
- Pus formation

Wound Management

Abrasions

Outer layers of skin are damaged from being scraped on a hard surface. Infection can occur and bleeding is limited due to the rupture of small veins and capillaries.

Initial care. Put on disposable latex gloves and follow OSHA guidelines. Using sterile gauze, cleanse affected area with soap and water to scrub particles out of the wound. After applying antibacterial ointment to the affected area, place dressing on affected area and cover with bandage.

Follow-up care. Change dressing daily and observe for signs of infection. Keep the wound moist with topical ointment so that the wound will heal from the inside out.

Avulsions

A forcible separation or tearing of tissue from the body in which bleeding occurs immediately.

Initial care. Put on disposable latex gloves and follow OSHA guidelines. Apply direct pressure with sterile gauze, elevate affected anatomical structure, watch for severe bleeding, and transport the athlete to a physician. Medical referral is required. Wrap the avulsed body part in a sterile gauze pad and place the body part in a plastic container of sterile water and ice.

Follow-up care. Follow the physician's directions in changing dressings and watch for signs of infection.

Laceration

A jagged, irregular tear in the soft tissues.

Initial care. Put on disposable latex gloves and follow OSHA guidelines. Using sterile gauze, cleanse area with soap and water to scrub particles out of the wound. Apply sterile gauze and direct pressure, elevate affected anatomical structure, watch for severe bleeding, and transport the athlete to a physician. Medical referral is recommended.

Follow-up care. Follow the physician's directions in changing the dressings and watch for signs of infection.

Puncture

A small hole in the tissues produced by an object (such as a nail) piercing the skin layers. External bleeding is limited, however internal damage to organs may cause bleeding.

Initial care. Put on disposable latex gloves and follow OSHA guidelines. Using sterile gauze, cleanse area with soap and water to scrub particles out of wound. Medical referral is recommended.

Follow-up care. Follow the physician's directions in changing the dressings and watch for signs of infection.

Management of Blisters

Blisters develop with friction to an area of the body, typically the foot or hand. Fluid accumulates under the skin and this is the body's attempt to reduce the friction to the area. If blood vessels are broken, there will also be an accumulation of blood in the blister; those are called blood blisters. Management of a blister usually depends on whether or not the blister is still intact. If the blister is intact, there are two schools of thought on the treatment. One, protect the area with a pad and allow the fluid to re-absorb into the body. This reduces the chance of infection and therefore the blister is not opened. The second school of thought is to open the blister, draining the fluid, and then protect it from infection and getting bigger. If the blister has ripped open, the standard treatment is to remove as much of the dead skin as possible, apply an antibacterial ointment to the area, and protect the area with a pad.

Management of Calluses

Calluses are formed over a period of time and typically on the foot or hand where the bone is right underneath the skin. This is done to toughen up the skin. Small callus formation is beneficial but excessive formation is counter productive. The standard treatment of an existing callus is to daily remove some of the skin with a callus remover (sand paper can be used) and then apply a skin-softener type lotion to keep the skin from drying out. Do not remove too much of the callus on any one day, but work on it daily and never use a knife to cut the callus off, this usually results in digging too deep and cutting into the skin and causing bleeding to occur.

Management of Laceration with Steri-Strip

A laceration is a rip to the skin, typically in an area where the bone is right under the skin as an example over the eye brow or chin area of the face. This type of injury can be treated with a specialized product called a steri-strip. This product is applied over the wound to close the wound and this will reduce the amount of scarring and speed up the healing process. This product can also be utilized on the field as a temporary wound care management until the athlete can be transported to a medical facility to receive stitches to close the wound.

Skin Conditions

There are a number of skin conditions that the athletic trainer or coach will be exposed to during a typical sport season. These conditions will range from very minor to the medical emergency. The establishment of appropriate protocol for the handling of all skin conditions will make your job easier and the care given to your athletes more complete. As with all conditions in which bodily fluids are present, you need to utilize latex gloves and follow the set of universal precautions in order to safeguard yourself in these matters. Additionally, the disposal of biohazardous waste must be done according to accepted guidelines of the local, state, and federal agencies. Following universal precautions for dealing with bodily fluids will help protect the athletic trainer and coach from disease or infection.

Methicillin-resistant *Staphylococcus Aureus* (MRSA) infections. MRSA is a type of staph bacteria that has become resistant to many of the antibiotic medications typically used to treat staph infections. Both traditional staph and MRSA can cause serious and even life threatening infections. These types of bacteria can be transmitted directly or indirectly from an infected person to an uninfected person. Direct transmission is usually in the form of direct person-to-person contact, which is common in many sport activities. Indirect transmission can occur from shared personal items (clothing, towels, razors) or shared athletic equipment. Early recognition and referring to proper healthcare providers for these skin infections is critical in successful management and treatment. Prevention is a critical component for reducing the risk of both traditional staph infections and MRSA infection. Practicing good personal hygiene is the best first step in prevention.

Recommendations from the Official Statement from the National Athletic Trainers' Association on Community-Acquired MRSA Infections (CA-MRSA)

Proper prevention and management recommendations may include, but are not limited to the following:

1. Keep hands clean by washing thoroughly with soap and warm water or using an alcohol-based hand sanitizer routinely.
2. Encourage immediate showering following activity.
3. Avoid whirlpools or common tubs if there are open wounds, scrapes, or scratches.
4. Avoid sharing towels, razors, and daily athletic gear.
5. Properly wash athletic gear and towels after each use.
6. Maintain clean facilities and equipment.
7. Inform or refer to appropriate health care personnel for all active skin lesions and lesions that do not respond to initial therapy.
8. Administer or seek proper first aid.
9. Encourage health care personnel to seek bacterial cultures to establish a diagnosis.
10. Care and cover skin lesions appropriately before participation.

Herpes simplex. A common problem in sports, particularly among wrestlers, is the skin infection called herpes simplex. The virus, which can enter the body through breaks in the skin, can produce painful lesions anywhere on the body. Most often, a lesion will appear as a cold sore on the lip. Even after the disease subsides, the athlete will continue to be a carrier of the virus and will be susceptible to future attacks. The danger of skin diseases such as herpes simplex is that they are highly contagious and can spread easily and rapidly to other members of the team. Another skin infection, impetigo, is similar in appearance to herpes simplex, but is much more contagious. Treatment and isolation can help prevent the infection of other athletes. The student athletic trainer should look for skin lesions on athletes. If they exist, medical referral to a physician is requested and you should advise the coaching staff to keep equipment (especially wrestling mats) clean and disinfected.

Fungus infections. Athlete's Foot (*Tinea Pedis*) The spread of athlete's foot depends mainly on the individual athlete's susceptibility. But, as a team, your athletes can help prevent athlete's foot from spreading by following this program:

- Powder the feet daily, using a standard fungicide.
- Dry the feet thoroughly after every shower, especially between and under the toes.
- Keep athletic shoes and street shoes dry by dusting them with powder daily.
- Wear clean sports socks and street socks daily.
- The shower and dressing rooms should be cleaned and disinfected daily.
- Athletes should use shower shoes. Once the tinea pedis fungus has infected an athlete, basic care includes the following:
  - Keep the feet as dry as possible through the frequent use of foot powder.
  - Wear clean, sports socks to avoid re-infection, changing them daily.
  - Use specific medicated fungicide.

Jock itch (*Tinea Cruris*). Jock itch may be due to an actual fungal infection. Other conditions referred to as "jock itch" can result from an accumulation of moisture in the groin area or from the friction of athletic activity. Jock itch appears as a brownish or reddish lesion in the groin area. The symptoms are mild to moderate itching, resulting in scratching and the possibility of a secondary bacterial infection. Direct contact, contaminated clothing or unsanitary locker rooms and showers may spread the contagious spores of this fungus. This fungus grows best in warm, moist, dark areas. If infected, this fungus can cause irritation to the athlete. The best ways to prevent jock itch are to keep the area clean and dry and to use a lubricating ointment to lessen friction in the groin area. Powders, sprays, and creams are used for treating jock itch but avoid medications that are irritating or tend to mask the symptoms of a groin infection. Infections that do not respond to normal treatment should be referred to the team physician.

Summary

Health care providers must not only take care of individuals, but should also safeguard themselves. Proper techniques and knowledge of the blood-borne pathogen guidelines will help to insure that infection and transmission of disease will be kept to a minimum. OSHA and CDC has taken the lead in providing the concepts to insure the safety of the health care professional and each institution must make sure that those precautions are known and followed.

References

Acello, B. (2002). *The OSHA handbook: The guidelines for compliance in healthcare facilities.* Clifton Park, NY: Thomas Delmar Learning.

American Medical Society for Sports Medicine and American Academy of Sports Medicine. (1995). Human immunodeficiency virus (HIV) and other blood-borne pathogens in sports. *American Journal of Sports Medicine, 23*(4), 510-514.

Center for Disease Control. (1995). Guidelines for prevention of transmission of human immunodeficiency virus and Hepatitis B virus to health-care and public workers. *Morbidity and Mortality Weekly Report.* Atlanta, GA.

Cohn, S., Dea, R., & Cooper, T. (2003). HIPAA: What's True, What Isn't. *The Permanente Journal.* Retrieved from http://xnet.kp.org/permanentejournal/sum03/hipaa.html

France,. R (2010). *Introduction to sports medicine and athletic training* (2nd ed.). Thomas Delmar Learning.

Glazer, J. (2002). Laceration Care. *Physician and Sports Medicine, 30*(7), 50.

Irion, G. (2009). *Comprehensive wound management* (2nd ed.). Thorofare, NJ: Slack, Inc.

Kohl, T., Martin, D., Nemeth, R., Evans, D., & Berks County Scholastic Athletic Trainers' Association. (2000). Wrestling Mats: Are They a Source of Ringworm Infection? *Journal of Athletic Training 35*,(4) pp. 427-430.

Kosan, L. (2006). *OSHA guidebook for labs* (2nd ed.). Marblehead, MA: HC Pro, Inc.

National Athletic Trainers' Association Board of Directors. (1995). Bloodborne pathogens for athletic trainers. *Journal of Athletic Training, 30*(3), 203-204.

National Federation of State High School Associations (NFHS) Sports Medicine Advisory Committee (2007). *MRSA in Sports Participation Position Statement and Guidelines.*

National Safety Council. (2003). *Blood-borne pathogens.* Boston, MA: Jones and Bartlett.

Occupational Safety and Health Organization. (1992). *Occupational exposures to blood-borne pathogens.* Washington, DC: United States Government Printing Office.

OSHA Fact Sheet. (2011). Blood-borne Pathogen Standard. Retrieved from www.osha.gov/OshDoc/data_BloodborneFacts/bbfact01.pdf

OSHA Fact Sheet. (2011). Bloodborne Pathogen Exposure Incidents. Retrieved from www.osha.gov/OshDoc/data_BloodborneFacts/bbfact04.pdf

Rankin, J., & Ingersoll, C. (2005). *Athletic training management concepts and applications* (3rd ed.). Boston, MA: McGraw-Hill.

Ray, R. (2011). *Management strategies in athletic training* (4th ed.). Champaign, IL: Human Kinetics.

Stockard, A. (2005). Methicillin-resistant staphylococcal aureas skin infection in athletes. *Texas Coach, 49*(7), pp. 42-44.

Van Ost, L., & Manfre, K. (2009). *Athletic training exam review: Student guide to success* (4th ed.). Thorofare, NJ: Slack Incorporated.

Winterstein, A. (2009). *Athletic training student primer: A foundation for success* (2nd ed.) Thorofare, NJ: Slack Incorporated.

World Wide Web: CDC, Diseases and Organisms in Healthcare Settings www.cdc.gov/HAI/organisms/organisms.html , Accessed March 4, 2013.

World Wide Web: CDC, Hepatitis B Information for the Public http://www.cdc.gov/hepatitis/B/index.htm, Accessed March 4, 2013.

World Wide Web: CDC, Methicillin-resistant Staphylococcus Aureus (MRSA) Infections http://www.cdc.gov/mrsa/, Accessed March 4, 2013.

World Wide Web: National Athletic Trainers' Association , Official Statement from the National Athletic Trainers' Association on Community-Acquired MRSA Infections (CA-MRSA) http://www.nata.org/sites/default/files/MRSA.pdf, Accessed March 4, 2013.

Review Questions

Completion

1. Wounds affect the_____, also known as the integument system.

2. In all follow-up wound care, the athletic trainer should look for signs of_____.

3. All soiled material should be placed in a_____.

4. OSHA guidelines cover bloodborne pathogens such as_____and_____.

5. The CDC estimates about_____infections occur each year of Hepatitis B.

6. A_____is when the outer layer of skin is scraped or scratched.

7. A sharp object causes an_____or_____wound.

8. Most fungus infections grow in an environment that is_____, _____, and_____.

Short Answer

1. List the five types of wounds mentioned in this chapter.

2. What is the difference between a laceration vs. avulsion?

3. What are the blood-borne pathogens that are of most concern in today's health care?

4. What solution is used to clean a contaminated athletic training room area?

5. How long does the bleach/water solution keep its effectiveness?

6. List the initial care for an avulsion.

7. Why is it important to have a plan of action to deal with blood-borne pathogens?

8. Why is herpes simplex a serious skin disease within an athletic team?

9. How would you care for athlete's foot?

5 Preventive and Supportive Techniques

Educational Objectives

Upon completing this chapter, the reader will be able to do the following:
- Describe the purpose and philosophy of taping and wrapping
- Identify the guidelines for the application of elastic wraps
- Identify the protocol in preparation of taping and/or wrapping
- Recognize the proper selection of supplies and equipment
- Recognize the precautions taken in the application of preventive/supportive techniques
- Recognize the importance of proper injury evaluation prior to application of preventive/supportive techniques
- Identify the proper steps in the application and removal of taping procedures

Assessing an Injury

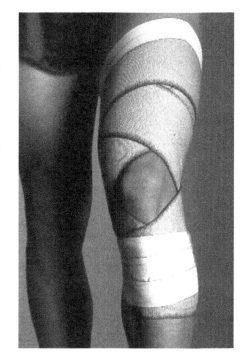

Before applying a preventive or supportive technique, a proper injury evaluation should be completed by a physician or qualified health care professional. If questions arise, a physician should perform a medical diagnosis. Following injury evaluation, a qualified health care professional can then make recommendations concerning application of protective techniques. This helps ensure that proper wrapping techniques are applied for support and stabilization. Also, it is imperative that the health care professional develop a thorough knowledge of wrapping and taping application fundamentals. While the basic principles of taping and wrapping are presented in this chapter, the learner should consult textbooks for a comprehensive description of taping and wrapping techniques.

Purpose of Taping and Wrapping

The primary purpose for tape application is to provide additional support, stability, and compression for the affected body part. The purpose of elastic wraps is for support and compression. Through proper application, taping and wrapping techniques can be applied to do the following:
- Shorten the muscles angle of pull
- Decrease joint range of motion
- Secure pads, bandages and protective devices
- Apply compression to aid in controlling swelling

Philosophy of Elastic Tape and Elastic Wrap Application

With tape application, proper angle, direction, and tension must be considered. Elastic tape has the ability to contract and expand and is commonly used in areas that need greater freedom of movement. Elastic tape also has the characteristics of conformability and strength. Additionally, it can be placed on the body part with fewer wrinkles and at greater angles. When applying elastic tape, proper tension must be applied.

Elastic wraps are primarily utilized in the application of applying either compression or support to injured anatomical structures. It is left to the discretion of the health care professional to select adhesive or elastic tape, and elastic wraps in the application of any preventive technique.

Common Terminology

- **Anchor**—anything that makes stable or secure, anything that is depended upon for support or security
- **Butterfly**—strips of tape that overlaps, as in "X" pattern
- **Check rein**—reinforced tape to restrict motion or movement
- **Collateral**—meaning side, lateral, and medial
- **Compression**—the act of applying pressure to a body part (i.e., applying a wrap, beginning at the bottom of an injury and wrapping toward the heart)
- **Diagonally**—a slanted or oblique direction
- **Diamond shape**—an object that is in the shape of two equilateral triangles placed base to base
- **Extension wrap**—a wrap used to assist in the extension of a specific joint
- **Figure of eight**—the bandaging of a joint where the initial turn circles the one part of the joint and the second turn circles the adjoining part of the joint to form a figure of eight
- **Flexion wrap**—a wrap used to assist in the flexion of that joint
- **Horizontal strip**—a strip that is placed level with the horizon, opposed to vertical strip
- **Horseshoe**—padding made to resemble the "U" shape
- **Hot spot**—early redness of the skin from friction that leads to a blister formation if preventive measures are not taken
- **Muscle contracted**—the shortening of the muscle
- **PRICES**—Protection, Rest, Ice, Compression, Elevation, and Support
- **Pad support**—a pad placed in a certain area to sustain, hold up, or maintain a desired position
- **Prophylactic**—denoting something that is preventative or protective
- **Shorten the angle of pull**—decreasing the range of motion of a joint
- **Spica wrap**—a figure eight bandage that generally overlaps the previous to form V like designs; used to give support, apply pressure or hold a dressing
- **Spiral**—applying a bandage around a limb that ascends the body part overlapping the previous bandage
- **Stirrup**—any "U" shaped loop or piece
- **Support**—to sustain, hold up or maintain a desired position
- **Swelling**—an increase in size of an area due to an increase in fluid
- **Tape mass**—adhesive applied to the cloth comprised of natural synthetic, zinc oxide, etc.
- **Vertical strip**—a strip that is placed perpendicular to the line of the horizon, opposed to horizontal strip
- **X-pattern**—the crossing of two pieces of tape in the shape of an X

Description of Athletic Training Supplies

The terminology of choice for this text will be adhesive tape or elastic tape. The adhesive tape is traditionally marketed as nonelastic, white tape. Elastic tape provides greater freedom of mobility to the affected body part, and is marketed as elastic tape. Both adhesive tape and elastic tapes are produced in a variety of widths. The terminology for elastic wrap is defined as a woven fabric that also allows for expansion and contraction, and is used for compression or supportive techniques. Elastic wraps are manufactured in 1", 2", 3", 4", and 6" widths, as well as double length. The ankle cloth wrap is nonelastic cloth that is 1 1/2" wide and between 72 - 96" in length. Additionally, adhesive and elastic tape is utilized to secure a wrap. In the preparation of some body parts, skin protection such as adhesive bandage with a lubricant must be considered.

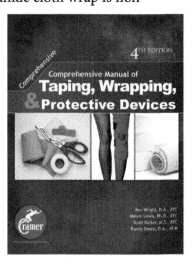

Selection of Proper Supplies and Specialty Supplies

One of the most critical aspects of taping techniques is the selection of proper supplies. Your selection depends on the number and types of sports offered and frequency of injuries. Purchasing supplies depends on budget, philosophy of medical staff regarding taping techniques, and occurrence of injury. Special consideration must be given to these additional supplies: benzoin (spray adherent), adhesive versus elastic tape, width of adhesive tape and elastic tape, and length and width of elastic wraps.

Preparation of Body Part to Be Taped or Wrapped

In preparing the body for taping and wrapping application, consider these items:
- **Removal of hair:** The athlete should shave the affected body part. This will ensure a good solid foundation for the tape, will allow for easy tape removal, and will reduce skin irritation.
- **Cleanse the area:** After hair removal, make sure the skin is clean and moisture free.
- **Special considerations:** Skin protection is important. Provide special care if the skin has any of the following: allergies, infections, open wounds, closed wounds, tape or tape adherent.
- **Spray adherent:** Spray the affected area with an adherent to aid in the adhesive quality.
- **Skin lubricants:** In areas of high friction or sensitivity, such as the Achilles tendon and the dorsum of the foot, a skin lubricant such as a heel and lace pad will help reduce the possibility of irritation.
- **Underwrap:** This foam wrap is used when the athlete is allergic to tape and/or to improve compliance. Foam wrap may also be used to hold heel and lace pads in place at high friction areas. The use of underwrap over the entire taping area can compromise the stability of the taping technique. When applying an elastic wrap, underwrap material should not be utilized.

Application and Removal of Taping Procedures

To tear tape, the adhesive tape is held firmly on each side of the proposed tear line. With proper tension applied on the tape, the free end is pulled away at an angle so that the force crosses the lines of the fabric of the backcloth at a sharp angle. The tear then occurs sequentially through the backcloth. The more quickly this maneuver is done, the more evenly tape edges will be torn. Some brands of elastic tape are extremely hard to tear by hand. Cut those brands with scissors to ensure proper tape application and neatness.

Easy removal of adhesive white tape and elastic tape is accomplished by using bandage scissors or a specially constructed tape cutter. A small amount of lubricant on the tip of the cutting device will allow the instrument to slip under the tape more readily, thus allowing removal of the tape with ease. Avoiding bony prominences, move the scissors or cutter along the natural channels or in areas of greatest soft tissue cushion.

Once this has been completed, remove the tape from the skin in a constant and gradual manner. It is preferred that the tape be removed in the opposite direction from which it was applied. When pulling the tape from the skin at an angle of 180 degrees, care should be exercised to minimize removal of skin tissue and skin irritation. It is recommended that pressure be applied to the skin (pull the skin away from the tape), to reduce the possibility of skin irritation. The daily use of a tape remover is recommended to help keep the skin clean and to prevent skin irritations and/or infections. Tape remover and/or alcohol will aid in the removal of tape mass and adherent from the skin. Following removal of tape, and post activity showering, lotion should be applied to the area that was taped.

Purpose and Application of Elastic Wraps for Support

During physical activity, supportive wraps are utilized to aid in muscle function and support and to reduce excessive range of motion. These applications are usually used for short periods, typically for competition or practice. Common terminology for these wraps are spica, figure of eight, and pad support. Spica wraps are traditionally employed at the hip and shoulder joints. Figure of eight wraps are placed over ankle, knee, elbow, and wrist and hand joints. Supportive wraps aid in securing pads after the proper placement of felt, foam rubber, and protective devices.

Purpose and Application of Elastic Wraps for Compression

Compression wraps are utilized in initial injury treatment protocol: Protection, Rest, Ice, Compression, Elevation, and Support (PRICES). In applying a compression wrap, use a spiral pattern, and, beginning distal to the injury, cross the injured joint, and finish proximal to the affected area. This combined with elevation, assists in moving fluids out of the injured area. In certain situations, it is preferred that the wrap start below the next joint. As with any wrapping procedure, removal and reapplication of compression wraps should take place every four hours.

Sport-Specific Rules on Taping and Wrapping

If you apply supportive techniques to an athlete, you should be aware of specific rules for that particular sport governing body has regarding tape and/or wrap applications. Your application must fall within the guidelines established for each sport by appropriate governing bodies.

Braces and Special Devices

The primary purpose for a protective device is to prevent an injury and to protect injured anatomical structures from further aggravation. Through proper application, a protective device can be applied to add additional protection, support, stability, and compression. The use of braces and special devices are beneficial if they are intelligently selected, used in the appropriate setting, correctly fitted, properly applied, and used within the rules and guidelines of the specific sport. Physician approval must be obtained prior to application and usage. Listed next are three common specialty supplies utilized in braces and special devices techniques.

Foam

Whether adhesive or nonadhesive, foam can be used in conjunction with various taping/wrapping procedures to increase efficacy of the technique. These items should be kept in mind when applying foam: proper size, thickness, shape, and foam composition needs to be determined prior to the application of the tape or wrap.

Thermoplastic

This rigid material can allow the injured athlete to return to practice and/or competition with an increased awareness that the injury will be protected from further harm. Because of the hard composition of this product, thermoplastic material may be restricted from some sports, limited to a certain body part, or require padding according to the guidelines of each sport.

Felt

This product should be applied with many of the same considerations as with foam rubber products. Factors that should be considered in the construction and application of a felt pad are size, thickness, and use of either adhesive or nonadhesive felt:

In the construction of a special pad, the following criteria should be considered.

1. Does the pad meet specific rules and guidelines of the sport? If NO, then do not use the pad.
2. Does the pad perform the function for which it was designed? If NO, then do not use the pad.
3. Will the pad contribute to further injury to the area or to an adjacent area? If YES, then do not use the pad.
4. Will the pad alter the function or void the warranty of a manufactured piece of equipment (i.e., helmet, shoulder pads)? If YES, then do not use the pad.

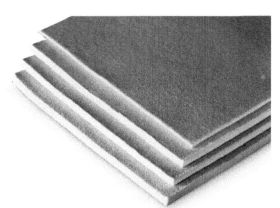

These and other common questions should routinely be asked and then answered by the health care professional before the construction of any specialty pad.

Principles of Physical Rehabilitation

Supportive techniques along with a rehabilitation program enhance an athlete's return to activity. Please note that taping and wrapping procedures are NOT a substitute for proper injury rehabilitation. You should follow specific instructions regarding injury rehabilitation and supportive taping techniques, as outlined by a physician or qualified health care professional. It is imperative that you as a health care professional develop a thorough knowledge of taping and wrapping application fundamentals.

Precautions

Before applying any technique, the athlete's skin temperature should be normal. To reduce the chance of skin irritation after any therapeutic treatment, allow adequate time for the skin to return to its normal temperature. This reduces the chance of skin irritation. When applying support techniques, the safety of the athlete should be your priority. Improper tape application can cause further injury. With all injured athletes, consultation with a physician is recommended. Tape application should not be used to allow participation with any disabling conditions.

Tips from the Field

- Know what body part and injury you are providing support and/or compression.
- Cover sensitive body parts (nail/nipple) and wounds with a protective covering.
- When applying a technique, learn to tape from a stationary position.
- Position the body part to be taped at your elbow height.
- When practicing, start with small length and width elastic wraps so you can learn common techniques like figure of eight, joint spica, etc. Once you are proficient with wraps, then utilize adhesive tape and elastic tape.
- Apply proper tension to the tape/wrap so that circulation will not be restricted.
- Follow the tape/wrap with your hand to smooth out all wrinkles.
- Overlap tape/wrap one-half its width to avoid spaces that could cause cuts and friction burns.
- When applying a compression wrap, always start distally and wrap proximally (toward the heart).
- Always angle tape in order for the tape ends to meet at the anchor strips. If you do not succeed, retry the angle at a sharper degree.
- When applying closure strips, it is recommended to always apply closure strips proximal to distal.
- When applying tape to the foot or ankle, pull the tape lateral to avoid excessive tension/ compression on the 5th metatarsal area.
- PRACTICE.

Preventive/Supportive Techniques

While basic taping and wrapping techniques are listed next, the learner should consult this chapter's reference list for texts that address comprehensive descriptions of taping and wrapping techniques.

Wrapping Techniques for Compression
Ankle compression wrap
Knee compression wrap
Elbow compression wrap
Wrist/hand compression wrap

Wrapping Techniques for Support
Ankle cloth wrap
Knee joint wrap
Hamstrings wrap
Quadriceps wrap
Hip flexor wrap
Hip adductor wrap
Glenohumeral joint wrap

Taping Techniques for the Ankle, Foot, and Lower Leg
Great toe
Heel
Metatarsal arch pad

Medial longitudinal arch
Toe splint
Plantar fasciitis
Ankle
Ankle: open basket weave
Shin splints
Achilles tendon

Taping Techniques for the Knee, Thigh, and Hip
Collateral knee
Hyperextended knee
Anterior cruciate
Patella tendon
Hip pointer

Taping Techniques for the Thorax and Low Back
Rib
Low Back

Taping Techniques for the Shoulder and Elbow
Acromioclavicular joint
Glenohumeral joint
Elbow hyperextended
Elbow epicondylitis

Taping Techniques for the Forearm, Wrist, and Hand
Forearm splint
Wrist
Thumb spica
Thumb c-lock
Finger splint
Collateral interphalangeal joint
Hyperextension of phalanges
Contusion to hand

Summary

Prophylactic taping, wrapping, and bracing must be done with proper application techniques, under the auspices of the physician or qualified health care professional, and must provide the proper biomechanical support and or stabilization. When done under those guidelines, the athlete can return to practice and competition quickly and safely. The physical structures of the human body can be assisted by the application of tape, wraps and braces. However, understand that taping and wrapping techniques are no substitute for proper conditioning and rehabilitation, but are very effective when used in conjunction with a program to prevent re-injury and expedite the healing and rehabilitation process.

References

Cerney, J. (1972). *Complete book of athletic taping techniques.* West Nyack, NY: Parker Publishing Inc.

Johnson & Johnson Consumer Products, Inc. (1993) *Athletic uses of adhesive tape* (1455 AD274), Skillman, NJ: Johnson & Johnson Consumer Products, Inc.

McDonald, R. (2010). *Pocketbook of taping techniques: Principles and practice.* London, UK: Churchill Livingstone Elsevier.

McDonald, R. (2004). *Taping techniques: Principles and practice,* (2nd ed.). Oxford, UK: Butterworth-Heinemann.

Miller, R., & Dunn, R. (1979*). Athletic training techniques.* Bowling Green, KY: WKU Press.

Street, S., & Rumkle, D. (2000). *Athletic protective equipment: Care, selection, and fitting.* St. Louis, MO: McGraw-Hill Higher Education.

Taber's Cyclopedic Medical Dictionary (22nd ed.). (2012). Philadelphia, PA: F. A. Davis.

Thompson, C., & Floyd, R. (2005). *Manual of structural kinesiology.* St. Louis, MO: McGraw-Hill higher Education.

Wright, K., Whitehill, W., & Lewis, M. (2005). *Preventive techniques: Taping/wrapping techniques and protective devices.* Gardner, KS: Cramer Products.

Wright, K., & Whitehill, W. (1996). *The comprehensive manual of taping and wrapping techniques* (2nd ed.) Gardner, KS: Cramer Products.

Wright, K., & Whitehill, W. (1991). *The comprehensive manual of taping and wrapping techniques.* Gardner, KS: Cramer Products

Suggested Multimedia Resources

Wright, K., & Whitehill. W. (1996). Sports Medicine Taping Series (Six Videos: *The Ankle; The Foot and Lower Leg; The Knee; The Shoulder and Elbow; The Wrist and Hand; Wrapping Techniques for Support & Compression*). St. Louis, MO: McGraw-Hill Higher Education.

Review Questions

Completion

1. Elastic tape has the ability to _____ and _____.

2. _____ is used in the initial treatment of acute injuries.

3. Proper skin temperature reduces the chances of _____.

4. Taping and wrapping procedures are not a substitute for proper _____.

Short Answer

1. What is the primary purpose of tape or elastic wraps?

2. How is a compression wrap applied?

3. In preparation of some body parts for applying tape, what would be applied for protection of the skin?

4. What is the importance of skin lubricants?

5. List three specialty supplies utilized in special pad techniques.

6. What should the skin temperature be for applying any taping technique?

7. Why should caution be used in the application of any taping and wrapping procedure?

8. What is the advantage of removing hair prior to applying a taping technique?

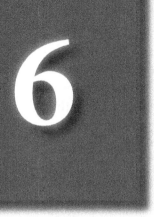

6 Foot, Ankle, and Lower Leg

Educational Objectives

Upon completing this chapter, the reader will be able to do the following:

- Name the anatomy of the foot, ankle and leg including bones, joints, muscles, and ligaments
- Identify the components of an evaluation format
- Compare the common injuries associated with the foot, ankle, and leg
- Demonstrate the principles of rehabilitation for the foot, ankle, and leg
- Describe the preventive/supportive techniques and protective devices for the lower extremity

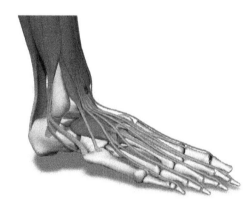

Anatomy

The foot is the site of some of the most minor, yet some of the most debilitating conditions suffered by athletes. Examples of these conditions include blisters, calluses, athlete's foot, turf toe, and ingrown toenails. Left untreated, these conditions can be just as disabling for an athlete as some of the more serious foot problems, such as heel bruises, arch strains, and fractures. The foot has stresses that exceed the demands placed on any other area of the body. The foot stabilizes and supports the rest of the body while standing, walking, running, or jumping. Whether the impact with the ground is on the heel, the ball of the foot, or the toes, the foot responds by absorbing several hundred pounds of force up to three times the body weight. Individually, the parts of the foot (bones, muscles, ligaments) are relatively weak. As a whole, however, the foot is strong enough to withstand most of the demands of athletics. The key to the foot's function is a set of four arches that help in absorbing the impact of walking, running, and jumping. The four arches of the foot are the metatarsal, transverse, medial (inner) longitudinal, and lateral (outer) longitudinal. The feet contain about one-fourth of the total number of bones in the body. Each foot has 26 bones (7 tarsal bones, 5 metatarsal, and 14 phalanges) and 38 joints. The tarsal bones are the talus, calcaneus, navicular, cuboid, and the medial, intermediate, and lateral cuneiform bones. The mid-foot region is made up of the 5 metatarsal bones. The toes have 14 bones known as the phalanges.

The talocrural joint (ankle joint) is the most commonly injured major joint in athletics. Fortunately, most injuries are either ligament sprains or muscular strains. Knowledge of the ankle's anatomy, its mechanism of injury, evaluation and first-aid procedures, preventive and supportive techniques are essential in reducing injury severity.

The talocrural joint is formed by three bones: tibia, fibula, and talus. Directly inferior to the talus is the calcaneus. The talus and the calcaneus form the subtalar joint. The tibia and fibula are the two bones of the lower leg, while the talus and calcaneus are the two largest bones of the foot. Those large, bony prominences (malleoli) on either side of the ankle are the distal ends of the tibia (medially) and the fibula (laterally).

The tibia, which transmits the weight or force placed on the lower leg to the talus, is mounted almost directly on top of the talus and extends over its medial side. On the lateral side of the talus the fibula extends, forming the lateral malleolus and helping to stabilize the ankle joint. The talocrural is a hinge joint with most of its movement in flexion (dorisflexion) and extension (plantarflexion), and the subtalar joint is triplanar with movement around an oblique axis where primarily the motions of inversion and eversion occur in the ankle. This joint is most stable when placed in dorsiflexion.

Covered by a layer of cartilage, the talus moves anteriorly (forward) and posteriorly (backward) in the cup-like cavity formed by the distal heads of the tibia and fibula. The talus acts as a movable saddle for the two bones of the lower leg. The talus, in turn, sits forward and on top of the calcaneus. The talus allows forward and downward movement of the ankle. The ankle joint, because of its arrangement of bones attaching ligaments, is structurally very strong. However, because of the stresses of athletics, the ankle is often injured. Since ankle injuries occur often, a comprehensive treatment and rehabilitation program must be followed prior to allowing an athlete to return to activity.

After the bony structure, the first line of defense against ankle sprains is the joint's strong ligamentous support. Just as with the bony structure, the ligaments of the ankle make the joint more stable medially. Most of the ligaments involved in supporting the ankle are attached to the rough edges of the malleoli. The ligaments are named for the bones they connect. The ligaments most commonly injured on the lateral aspect of the ankle are the anterior talofibular, calcaneofibular, and posterior talofibular. The anterior talofibular ligament is the most commonly sprained ligament in the body and is typically the first ligament to be sprained during a classic inversion mechanism of injury such as landing on someone's foot or stepping in a hole. On the medial aspect, the deltoid ligament is commonly injured. For evaluation purposes, the athletic training or coach should know the location of all the ankle joint ligaments.

Thirteen major muscles support the ankle joint. Two of the muscle tendon groups most important in preventing ankle injuries are the Achilles tendon and the peroneus muscle group. A tight Achilles tendon, which is the attachment of the gastrocnemius and soleus muscles (calf muscles) to the calcaneus, is often the cause of recurrent ankle sprains. The peroneal muscle group runs along the lateral side of the leg and foot, attaching at several areas on the foot. The peroneal brevis attaches on the lateral aspect of the foot, at the base of the fifth metatarsal whereas the peroneal longus runs across the plantar surface of the foot and inserts into the lateral base of the first metatarsal and medial cunneiform. When the peroneal group contracts, it causes the foot to evert, which helps to prevent a sprain to the lateral ligaments.

The two bones of the leg are the tibia and the fibula. The area on the front of the leg is called the shin, which includes the following muscles: tibialis anterior, extensor hallucis longus, and extensor digitorum longus. Often associated with shin pain is the interosseous membrane, which connects the tibia and fibula. On the posterior aspect of the leg are the gastrocnemius and soleus muscles, the Achilles tendon, and the tibialis posterior, flexor digitorum longus, and flexor hallucis longus. Often called the heel cord, the Achilles tendon of the calf muscles attaches to the calcaneus, or heel bone. This area of the body is innervated by a number of different nerves. The sensory distribution of a nerve root is called a dermatome, which produces sensation in a corresponding anatomical area. The motor distribution of a group of muscles innervated by a single nerve root is called a mytome and it produces movement of anatomical structures. Additionally, anatomical structures that can be injured include the fat pads, bursi and plantar fascia. Fat pads are specialized soft tissue structure for weight bearing and absorbing impact, whereas synovial sacs located over bony prominences throughout the body are called bursi.

Foot, Ankle, and Leg Anatomy

Bones
- Tibia
- Fibula
- Talus

- Calcaneus
- Navicular
- Cuneiforms (1-3)
- Cuboid
- Metatarsals (1-5)
- Phalanges (1-5)

Ligaments
- Plantar calcaneonavicular ligament
- Posterior talocalcaneal ligament
- Calcaneofibular ligament
- Calcaneonavicular ligament
- Lateral talocalcaneal ligament
- Anterior talofibular ligament
- Posterior talofibular ligament
- Deltoid ligament

Joints
- Talocrural (ankle)
- Metatarsophalangeal (MTP)
- Tarsometatarsal
- Intertarsal
  - Subtalar (talocalcaneal)
  - Talocalcaneonavicular
  - Calcaneocuboid
  - Talonavicular
  - Cuneonavicular
  - Cuneocuboid
- Interphalangeal (IP): proximal and distal

Muscles

To view videos and other materials related to this chapter on the FOOT, ANKLE, AND LOWER LEG, see access instructions on the last page of this text.

Table 6.1
Compartments, Muscles, and Actions of the Lower Leg

Compartment of Lower Leg	Muscle	Action
Anterior	Tibialis anterior	Dorsiflexion and inversion
	Extensor digitorum longus	Extension of toes 2-5
	Extensor hallucis longus	Extension of great toe
Lateral	Peroneus longus	Eversion and plantarflexion
	Peroneus brevis	Eversion and plantarflexion
Posterior	Gastrocnemius	Plantarflexion
	Soleus	Plantarflexion (with knee bent)
Deep Posterior	Tibialis posterior	Inversion and plantarflexion
	Flexor digitorum longus	Flexion of toes 2-5
	Flexor hallucis longus	Flexion of great toe

Arches
- Metatarsal
- Transverse
- Medial longitudinal (inner)
- Lateral longitudinal (outer)

Range of Motion
- **Dorsiflexion:** the act of drawing the toe or foot toward the dorsal aspect of the proximally conjoined body segment (decreasing angle between the top of the foot and leg).
- **Plantar flexion:** the act of drawing the toe or foot toward the plantar aspect of the proximally conjoined body segment (increasing angle between the top of the foot and leg).
- **Inversion:** turning the sole of the foot inward (subtalar/talocalcaneal joint movement)
- **Eversion:** turning the sole of the foot outward (subtalar/talocalcaneal joint movement)
- **Flexion (toes):** decreasing the angle between the toes and the sole of the foot
- **Extension (toes):** increasing the angle between the toes and the sole of the foot
- **Pronation:** combined motions of calcaneal eversion, foot abduction and dorsiflexion
- **Supination:** combined motions of calcaneal inversion, foot adduction and plantar flexion
- **Abduction:** movement of body segment away from midline of the body
- **Adduction:** movement of body segment toward the midline of the body

Dermatomes
L4—Anteriomedial aspect of lower leg and medial side of foot and great toe
L5—Dorsum of foot
S1—Lateral aspect of foot and distal posterior aspect of lower leg
S2—Proximal 1/3 of posterior aspect of lower leg

Myotomes
L4—Dorsiflexion of ankle
L5—Extensor hallucis longus, toe extension
S1—Plantar flexion of ankle or hamstring curl, foot eversion, hip extension
S2—Knee flexion

When determining the strength of myotomes, provide resistive force.

Evaluation Format

The first purpose of an evaluation is to determine if a serious injury has occurred. Initially, a fracture should always be suspected. Signs of a fracture include, but are not limited to, direct or indirect pain, deformity, or a grating sound at the injury site. Some fractures are not accompanied by swelling or pain. If a fracture is suspected, the extremity should be splinted and the athlete transported for medical evaluation. Young athletes are especially susceptible to fractures, due to their immature bone structure. Often, ligaments and muscles are stronger than the bones. The evaluation process to help determine the type of injury involves four steps: history, observation, palpation, and special tests.

(H) History
This involves asking questions of the athlete to help determine the mechanism of injury. Answers to these questions will help to adequately assess the injury and assist the certified athletic trainer or the physician in a diagnosis.
1. Mechanism of injury (How did it happen?)
2. Location of pain (Where does it hurt?)

3. Sensations experienced (Did you hear a pop or snap?)
4. Previous injury (Have you injured this anatomical structure before?)

(O) Observation

Compare the uninjured to the injured lower extremity and look for bleeding, deformity, swelling, discoloration, scars, and other signs of trauma.

(P) Palpation

Palpation is the physical inspection of an injury. First, palpate the anatomical structures/joints above and below the injuried site. Then palpate the affected area. The entire area around the injury may be sore, but the athletic training student or coach should try to pinpoint the site of severe pain. From knowledge of the lower extremity's anatomy and injury mechanism, the type and extent of injury can be evaluated. Involve the athlete in the evaluation as much as possible. Using bilateral comparison, these items should be palpated/performed:
1. Neurological (motor and sensory)
2. Circulation (pulse and capillary refill)
3. Anatomical structures (palpate)
4. Fracture test (palpation, compression, and distraction)

(S) Special Tests

With all special tests, the certified athletic trainer is looking for joint instability, disability, and pain. It is possible to further damage an injury through manipulation. These tests are well beyond the expertise of an athletic training student or coach. To determine if damage has been done to the anatomical structures, the certified athletic trainer uses special functional tests to assess disability. These include the following:
1. Joint stability (ligament)
2. Muscle/tendon
3. Accessory anatomical structures
4. Inflammatory conditions
5. Range of motion (active, assistive, passive and resistive)
6. Pain or weakness in the affected area.
7. Refer to Chapter 2 for a full explanation of the HOPS injury evaluation format.

Conditions that Indicate an Athlete Should Be Referred for Physician Evaluation

- Gross deformity
- Significant pain
- Increased swelling
- Circulation or neurological impairment
- Joint instability
- Suspected fracture or dislocation
- Abnormal sensations such as clicking, popping, grating, or weakness
- Persistant pain within the lower leg compartments
- Any doubt regarding the severity or nature of the injury

When an X-Ray Is Appropriate

In 1992, the Ottawa Ankle Rules were developed to assist emergency room physicians in determining whether a patient with an ankle or foot injury should receive an X-ray to determine if a fracture

was present. These rules have been modified since then and further research has shown these rules to be highly accurate in the decision to receive an X-ray (Bachmann, 2003). It is important to understand that if there is any doubt about the severity of an ankle injury, it is a best practice to refer to a physician or a certified athletic trainer for further consultation. The Ottawa Ankle Rules state that a patient should receive an X-ray for an ankle or foot if any one of the following conditions are true:
- Inability to walk four steps immediately after the injury
- Tenderness on the posterior edge or tip of the medial or lateral malleolus
- Tenderness on the navicular
- Tenderness on the base of the fifth metatarsal

Common Injuries

Ankle Sprains

Ankle injuries range from muscle strains and ligament sprains to dislocations and fractures. The most common injury is the sprain. The mechanism of injury for a lateral ankle sprain is usually a combination of excessive inversion and plantar flexion. The mechanism is similar to an athlete stepping into a hole or landing on another player's foot. More than 80% of all ankle sprains are of this type of mechanism. The ligament most often injured is the anterior talofibular ligament. Since most sprains are of the lateral, or inversion type, ankle tapings have been designed to prevent the inversion sprain. Less common is the eversion sprain. On the medial side of the ankle is the tough, thick deltoid ligament, which helps prevent excessive eversion or turning of the heel outward movement. A third type of ankle sprain is termed the "high" ankle sprain, which involves the anterior tibiofibular ligament which connects the tibia to the fibula. The mechanism of injury for a high ankle sprain is typically a combination of eversion and abduction of the foot.

Whether the sprain is of the inversion, eversion, or eversion/abduction type, it is usually placed into one of three categories: first degree (mild), second degree (moderate), or third degree (severe).

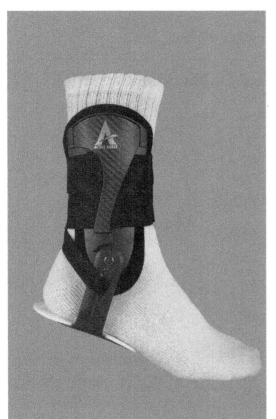

First degree sprain. In a first degree sprain, one or more of the supporting ligaments and surrounding tissues are stretched. There is minor discomfort, point tenderness, and little or no swelling. There is no abnormal movement in the joint to indicate lack of stability.

Second degree sprain. A second degree sprain happens when a portion of one or more ligaments is torn. There is pain, swelling, point tenderness, disability and loss of function. There is slight abnormal movement in the joint. The athlete may not be able to walk normally and will favor the injured leg.

Third degree sprain. In a third degree sprain, one or more ligaments have been completely torn, resulting in joint instability. There is either extreme pain or little pain (if nerve damage has occurred), loss of function, point tenderness, and rapid swelling. An accompanying fracture is possible.

While the procedures to determine the severity of the ankle sprain are best left to the certified athletic trainer or orthopedic physician, it is important to understand the proper treatment of an acute ankle sprain. An ice bag is the best modality to decrease the athlete's pain and to limit the amount of swelling that may occur. The ice bag should be wrapped onto the ankle for at least 20 minutes with an elastic wrap and the athlete should elevate their ankle above the heart to discourage swelling in the ankle. It is important to note that if a coach or player uses a chemical ice bag instead of the normal bag full of ice, then the treatment time should be no more than 15-20 minutes as the chance for a chemical burn of the athlete's skin is greatly increased with a chemical ice bag. The athlete should be referred to the certified athletic trainer or physician for proper determination of the exact injury and severity.

For an athlete with a lateral or medial ankle sprain, a horseshoe pad should be applied with an elastic wrap around the lateral malleolus (for lateral ankle sprain) or medial malleolus (for medial ankle sprain). This combination of an elastic wrap and horseshoe pad will further limit the amount of swelling that occurs in the athlete's ankle. If the athlete is unable to walk with correct form, then they should be fitted for crutches until seen by the athletic trainer or physician. The key to treating acute ankle sprains is to limit the amount of swelling in the injured area, the less swelling that accumulates, the less that needs to be removed before the athlete can initiate rehabilitation and return to play.

Blisters and Calluses

Although blisters can occur on any part of the body where friction exists, in athletics blisters are most often found on the feet. As the layers of the skin rub together, friction causes separation. The body responds with fluid formation in this separation. This fluid creates pressure on nerve endings, which is perceived as pain. If the blister is neglected, it may break, creating an open wound. Once formed, blisters cannot be ignored. Proper treatment of a blister is mandatory in order to ensure maximum comfort of the athlete and to reduce the possibility of infection. Blisters can be very painful and even debilitating if not properly treated. Proper treatment of a blister is dependent on the size and location of the blister in the foot and ankle. In general, if a blister breaks on its own, it is best to clean with soap and water, apply an antibacterial ointment, and cover the blister to keep clean and expedite the healing process. In addition, a doughnut pad may be applied to redistribute the friction to the pad instead of the injured area which decrease pain and limits further injury.

Calluses are areas of skin that are typically rougher and thicker than other adjacent areas of the foot that develop as the body's response to chronic friction in an area. For athletes who run, cut, and jump as part of their sport, it is normal to see calluses on the soles of the feet or along the toes. However, it is best to avoid a situation where calluses become too thick. When calluses become too thick, blisters can form underneath the callus. Blisters underneath a callus usually do not break on their own and therefore cause pain for an extended amount of time. It is best for the athlete to develop the habit of shaving down a callus so that it is only slightly thicker than the adjacent skin to avoid developing a blister underneath the callus.

Arch Sprains

Most people are unaware that there are four arches in the foot. Each contributes to balance, movement, support, and shock absorption. To help understand these arches, place a wet foot down on an absorbent paper towel and observe the footprint. Any of the four arches of the foot (transverse, metatarsal, inner, or outer longitudinal) can suffer supportive ligament The primary arch of the foot is the medial longitudinal arch, which is supported by the plantar calcaneonavicular ligament or "spring" ligament and the plantar fascia. Once the ligaments are stretched, they fail to hold the bones of the foot in position.

When an arch is weakened in this manner, it cannot absorb shock as well as it is designed to do. Resulting manifestations may include shin splints, Achilles tendon strain, foot fatigue, strained muscles, and even blisters. If the athletic training student or coach treats only the symptoms, the arch sprain may worsen. Causes of arch problems include overuse, overweight, fatigue, training on hard surfaces, and wearing nonsupportive, worn shoes. First aid, as with other ligament sprains, includes cold, compression, and elevation. Most arch sprains are to the metatarsal arch or inner longitudinal arch. A common sign of the metatarsal arch sprain is a callus that appears along the head of the third metatarsal indicating that the arch is falling.

Shin Splints (Medial Tibial Stress Syndrome)

The term *shin splints* has inaccurately become a catchall term to describe pain or injury of the anterior portion of the lower leg. The medical term for this condition is Medial Tibial Stress Syndrome. However, for the athletic training or coach to assume that any leg pain in athletics is a symptom of shin splints would be a mistake. Two other much more serious injuries often have similar symptoms to shin splints. These injuries are stress fractures and anterior compartment syndrome. The shin splint injury is thought to be an inflammation of the interosseous membrane, strains to the soleus muscle, or other chronic lower leg conditions. Because of the leg's poor blood supply, any injury in this region can be slow to heal. Shin splints have been attributed to tight deep posterior muscles, specifically the soleus and tibialis posterior, which become irritated due to decreased dorsiflexion and improper medial longitudinal arch support. Preferred treatment should include cryotherapy, foot support (orthotics), and medical referral. Left untreated and uncorrected, the condition can worsen until it is disabling. Some causes of shin splints are muscle weakness or imbalance, lack of proper conditioning, improper or incomplete warmup, poor flexibility or lack of stretching, running on hard surfaces, improper running form or habits, improper or worn running shoes, or poor support for anatomical structures. The focus of a typical rehabilitation plan include exercises designed to strengthen the muscles of the deep posterior compartment of the lower leg which help support the medial longitudinal arch.

Great Toe Sprain (Turf Toe)

The great toe is very important in balance, movement, and speed. Occasionally, the ligaments supporting the toe will become sprained, severely limiting the athlete's performance. Turf toe is the name given to such a sprain. Often, the mechanism of the injury will be the foot sliding back on a slippery surface, which forcefully hyperextends the toe. As with any acute sprain, immediate care of turf toe is protection, rest, ice, compression, elevation, and support. The physician may take X-rays to rule out a more severe injury. Most sprains of the great toe are minor, however since the normal walking/running motion requires great toe extension, a turf toe injury can become a chronic injury that may last most of a competitive season. Once normal function returns, the patient should be encouraged to have constant foot/toe support, such as a turf toe tape job, to prevent limit movement of the great toe. Perhaps one of the worst footwear choices an athlete can wear when recovering from a sprained great toe are flip-flops due to the lack of support and excessive motion in the joint when walking.

Plantar Fasciitis (Plantar Aponeurosis)

The plantar fascia is a wide, nonelastic ligamentous tissue that extends from the anterior portion of the calcaneus to the heads of the metatarsals, supplying support to the longitudinal arch of the foot. This tissue can become strained from overuse, unsupportive footwear, a tight Achilles tendon or running on hard surfaces. Most often, the cause of plantar fasciitis is chronic irritation. Cross-country and track athletes are prone to overuse injuries in which the plantar fascia is continually strained from running and jumping Basketball and volleyball athletes are also susceptible to plantar fasciitis from repeated jumping and landing. An athlete with plantar fasciitis will experience pain and tenderness on the bottom of the foot near the heel. A common complaint of the athlete with plantar fasciitis is increased pain when first walking in the morning after getting out of bed. This is due to the plantar fascia being in a shortened position (plantarflexion) during sleeping hours and then suddenly stretched during the first steps in the morning. Untreated, this condition causes bone imbalance which can lead to heel spurs, muscle strains, shin splints, and other problems. In addition to the basic treatment of ice and rest, arch supports (e.g., orthotics, arch taping, etc.) can provide additional relief of stress on the plantar fascia.

Heel Bruise

The heel receives, absorbs, and transfers much of the impact from sports activities, especially running and jumping. Therefore, the ligaments, tendons, and fat pad of the heel are all subject to stress and injury. The heel bruise is among the most disabling contusions in athletics. The heel must be protected during physical activity Cold application before activity, and cold and elevation afterwards can help reduce swelling and pain. To assist the patient, supply a heel cup to help absorb the force of the heel's impact with the ground or floor, or a donut pad can be constructed to protect the bruised area. In order to prevent muscle imbalance and problems from misalignment of the body, both shoes, not just the shoe of the injured foot, should contain equal amounts of padding.

Heel Spur

A heel spur is a bony growth on the calcaneus that causes painful inflammation of the accompanying soft tissue and is aggravated by exercise. The athlete can locate a heel spur by pressing on the heel. As the foot flattens, the plantar fascia is stretched and pulled at the point where it attaches to the calcaneus. Over a period of time, the calcaneus reacts to this irritation by forming a spur of bony material. The team physician may recommend taping the arch or using shoe inserts (orthoses) to help reduce the plantar fascia's pull on the calcaneus.

Anterior Compartment Syndrome

Anterior compartment syndrome is a condition that, when suspected by the coach or athletic training student, should be referred immediately to the physician. The four compartments of the lower leg are listed in Table 6.1.

Most compartment syndromes in athletics are to the anterior compartment. As with stress fractures, anterior compartment syndrome can be mistaken for shin splints. In addition, anterior compartment syndrome can be misdiagnosed as a contusion of the shin, muscle cramps, or spasms. The anterior compartment is tightly filled with the muscles that dorsiflex the foot and ankle. It is almost entirely enclosed with rigid walls of bone or tissue. Misdiagnosis of this condition could lead to permanent muscle tissue damage, resulting in permanent disability. Direct trauma or excessive exercise can result in hemorrhage and swelling inside the compartment. This swelling will increase the pressure on the deep peroneal nerve, the veins, and, finally, the arteries inside the compartment. Without arterial circulation, muscle cells will die. Signs of anterior compartment syndrome include pain even after cold treatment, a firmness of the muscle, numbness of the foot, and warmth. **Once suspected, anterior compartment syndrome should be treated as a medical emergency.**

Achilles Tendon Strain

Although the Achilles tendon is the strongest in the body, it is a vulnerable area for athletes. Severe damage, such as a tear, can be career-threatening. The tendon is formed by the union of the gastrocnemius and soleus muscles on the back of the leg. The tendon inserts on the calcaneus. Injuries can be caused by overuse, muscle inbalance, inflexibility, or a sudden movement. Depending on the force and the condition of the tendon, the injuries can range from mild strains to complete ruptures. Strains of this important tendon must be treated more conservatively with protection, rest, ice, compression, elevation, and support (PRICES) than most muscle injuries. This is because of the disability the injury produces and the tendency for the strain to develop into a complete tear. The Achilles tendon is sometimes strained when the ankle is sprained, and may take longer to heal than the injured ligaments. A strong and flexible Achilles tendon can prevent many ankle sprains.

Stress Fractures

Bones are not inanimate objects. They are living tissue. Just like muscle cells, bone cells respond to exercise, growing stronger to meet new demands. Lack of exercise can lead to deterioration or deossification of the bone. If the exercise is too severe, or of too long a duration, the change in the bone structure will be negative and a stress fracture can begin to develop. Continued stress will lead to a worsening of the fracture. Because stress fractures often occur in the lower extremity, there is a tendency to dismiss pain in this anatomical region. Early X-rays may not reveal evidence of the stress fracture, but after conversative treatment and rest, a second series of X-rays three to four weeks after the initial set of X-rays may be indicated to confirm or rule out stress fractures. Signs of a stress fracture might include specific point tenderness and increased pain during exercise sessions. Usually a stress fracture will hurt when the athlete presses with the fingers just above and below the site of most pain. In later stages of stress fractures, pain is constant, especially at night. If a stress fracture is suspected, medical referral is recommended.

One type of stress fracture is the March fracture, which typically occurs to the 2nd or 3rd metatarsal. This can be seen with any athlete who runs but most commonly seen with distance runners. This name is given because it was most commonly seen in soldiers who had to march great distances and developed these stress fractures. A march fracture typically develops due to a flattened metatarsal arch.

Muscle Cramps

In athletics, athletic trainers often see an athlete make a rapid recovery from what appears to be a painful, disabling knee or ankle injury. In those cases, the injury may simply be a cramp in the muscles of the lower extremity. A cramp is a sudden, involuntary contraction of a muscle. While the cause is unknown, several factors seem to contribute to their incidence:

- Fatigue
- Dehydration
- Lack of nutrients in diet
- Poor flexibility
- Previous injury, where rehabilitation program was not completed
- Improperly fitted equipment that causes excessive strain on the anatomical structure

Rehabilitation

Sending an athlete back to competition before healing is complete leaves the player susceptible to further injury. The best way to determine when healing is complete is by the absence of pain during stressful activity and by the return of full range of motion and strength, power, and endurance to the affected muscle group. Prior to the beginning of any rehabilitation exercise program, a coach should consult with the sports medicine team to establish an individual program tailored for that individual athlete and the specific injury to be rehabilitated. The following list of exercises can be used as rehabilitative or preventive exercises.

Range of Motion Exercises	Ankle
Dorsiflexion	Ankle alphabet
Plantar flexion	Heel raises
Inversion	Toe raises
Eversion	Incline board
Flexion (toes)	Mini squats
Extension (toes)	Proprioception exercises
Circumduction	
	Foot
Lower Leg	Sponge pick-ups
Heel raises	Marble pick-ups
Toe raises	Towel gathering

Included in any rehabilitation protocol is the following:
- Range of motion exercises
- Resistive exercises
- Cardiovascular/fitness activities (walking, squatting, stair climbing, progressive running, cycling)
- Sport-specific activities (jumping, figure of eights, jumping rope, etc.)

Return to Competition Guidelines

Before returning to competition, the following rehabilitation guidelines must be met:
- Full range of motion
- Strength, power, and endurance are proportional to the athlete's size and sport
- No pain during running, jumping, or cutting

Preventive/Supportive Techniques

The application of preventive and supportive techniques is a time-consuming tradition and can be a very expensive practice. Whether to apply adhesive and/or elastic bandages to an uninjured anatomical structure is a decision the certified athletic trainer will have to make. The taping technique listed below are fundamental procedures utilized to support various anatomical structures of the foot, ankle and leg. To increase your knowledge of additional techniques, please consult the texts listed in the appendix.

Wrapping Techniques for Compression
Ankle

Wrapping Techniques for Support
Ankle cloth

Taping Techniques for the Ankle, Foot, and Lower Leg
Great toe
Heel
Metatarsal arch pad
Medial longitudinal arch
Toe splint
Plantar fasciitis
Ankle
Ankle: Open basket weave
Shin splint
Achilles tendon

Protective Devices

The use of protective devices is beneficial, if they are properly selected, used in the appropriate setting, correctly fitted, and follow the guidelines of the specific sport. Consultation with an equipment specialist is highly encouraged. Listed below are various protective devices that are commercially available to use in sport:

- Achilles brace (Achilles tendons tendinitis straps)
- Ankle braces (lace-up, air, prophylactic, etc.)

- Arch supports
- Boots (hockey, ski, wrestling)
- Bunion pads
- Corn and callus pads
- Heel cups
- Heel lifts
- Orthosis (soft, semirigid, rigid)
- Shin guards
- Shoes (basketball, baseball, racing, running, golf, track, etc.)
- Shinsplint brace
- Turf toe brace

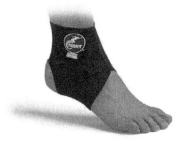

Muscoloskeletal Conditions/Disorders

The following is a list of other common musculoskeletal disorders that affect the foot, ankle, and leg. Consult with either *Tabers's Cyclopedic Medical Dictionary* or *Signs and Symptons of Athletic Injuries* for definitions of these terms.

- Apophysitis calcaneus
- Bunion (hallus valgus)
- Bunionette
- Bursitis
- Corn
- Exotoses
- Fractures (tibia, fibula, tarsals, metatarsals, phalanges)
- Hallux rigidus
- Hallux varus
- Hammer toe
- Interdigital neuroma

- Ingrown toenail
- Morton's syndrome
- Pes cavus
- Pes planus
- Plantar neuroma
- Sesamoiditis
- Superficial achilles bursitis
- Supple flatfoot
- Stone bruise
- Talotibial extosis
- Tarsal tunnel syndrome
- Tendinitis/tenosynovitis

Ankle Compression Wrap

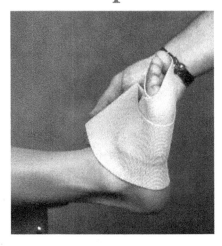 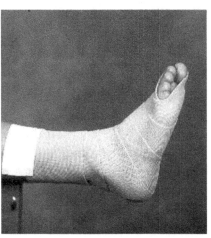

1. Begin the 4" elastic wrap at the distal part of the phalanges, spiral the wrap around the foot and ankle and on the distal aspect of the lower leg.
2. Secure the wrap with a small strip of 1 1/2" adhesive tape.

Ankle Taping

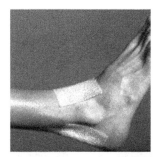
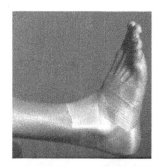

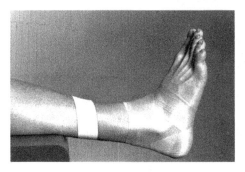
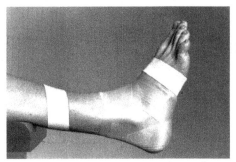
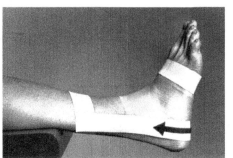

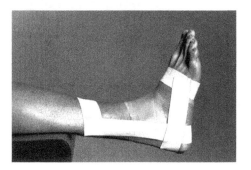
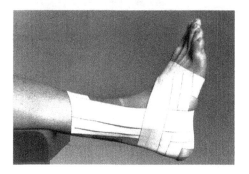

1. Apply an adhesive tape anchor strip around the lower leg at approximately the musculo-tendon junction of the gastrocnemius. Since the leg at this site is not cylindrically shaped, the tape must be angled slightly to conform to the leg.
2. Apply an additional anchor at the instep. Remember that excessive tension on the 5th metatarsal could cause pain upon weight bearing.
3. Apply the first of three stirrup strips. Beginning on the medial aspect of the upper anchor, this stirrup continues down the inside of the leg, over the medial malleolus, across the plantar aspect of the foot, over the lateral malleolus, up the lateral aspect of the leg, and ends at the lateral aspect of the upper anchor. Proper tension must be applied to cause some eversion of the foot, thus helping to reduce inversion.
4. Apply the first of three horse shoe strips. The first horizontal strip is started on the medial aspect of the foot, continues toward the heel and below the medial malleolus, crosses the Achilles tendon below the lateral malleolus, and ends on the lateral aspect of the foot.
5. Repeat steps #3 and #4 twice, overlapping the tape one-half its width. These interlocking strips should provide additional support for this technique. The completed portion of this closed basket weave has sets of interlocking stirrups and horse shoe strips. Apply a proximal anchor for support. For proper adherence, apply compression to the tape so that the tape conforms to the body part.

Ankle Taping

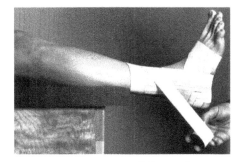 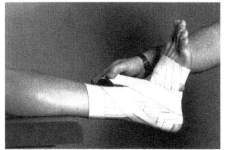 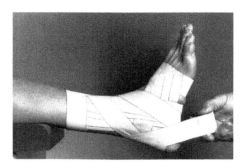

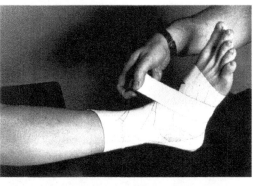 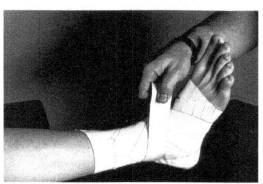

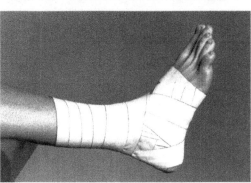 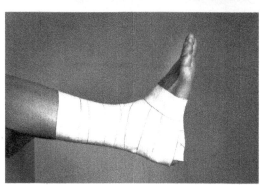

6. Apply the first heel lock strip. Begin on the anterior portion of the upper anchor. This **lateral heel lock** will continue down the outside of the leg, crossing the Achilles tendon, around the medial aspect of the heel, angling underneath the foot, and moving up the lateral aspect of the leg. Proper tension must be applied to insure stabilization of the calcaneus.

7. Apply the second heel lock strip. Begin on the anterior portion of the upper anchor. This **medial heel lock** will continue down the inside of the leg, crossing the Achilles tendon, around the lateral aspect of the heel, angling underneath the foot, and moving up the medial aspect of the leg.

8. A **figure of eight** is applied next. Starting on the dorsal aspect of the foot, move medially down the inside of the foot, across the plantar portion, up the outside of the foot to the starting point. Continuation of the tape will proceed medially around the lower leg crossing the Achilles tendon, and finishing at the origin of this figure of eight technique. By encircling the foot and lower leg, this technique will assist in dorsal flexion and eversion.

9. Final closure strips are then applied. Begin proximally and work distally. From the upper anchor, apply individual circular strips around the extremity to cover tape ends. Make sure you overlap the tape approximately one-half its width on each strip.

Great Toe

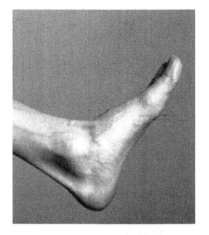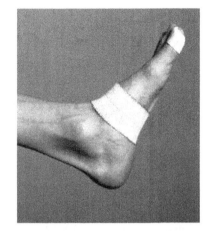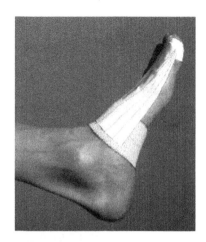

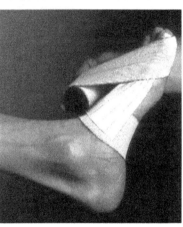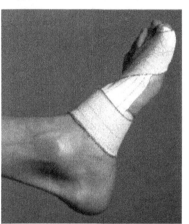

To begin the taping procedure, place the athlete's ankle and the first MP joint in a neutral position and cover the nail with a band-aid.

1. Apply two anchor strips.
   A) Apply adhesive anchor strip around distal aspect of the great toe.
   B) Apply elastic anchor strip around the mid-foot. This strip should begin on the dorsal aspect, go lateral, and continue across the plantar aspect to the mid-foot medial portion, crossing the tape ends.
2. Four to six strips of adhesive tape should be applied to form a fan shape. This will provide adequate support. Place fan-shaped tape from the anchor on the great toe, covering the affected area and ending on the elastic anchor at the mid-foot.
3. Using a continuous strip of elastic tape, apply a figure of eight around the great toe and mid-foot. This will aid in abduction of the first MP joint and should assist in preventing excessive movement, flexion or extension of the MP joint.

This adjunct taping procedure can be used in conjunction with the basic technique presented.

Technique A: Apply two circular strips of adhesive tape, around the proximal and distal aspect of first and second phalanges. This is commonly referred to as buddy taping.

References

American Academy of Orthopaedic Surgeons. (2000). *Athletic training and sports medicine.* Chicago, IL: American Academy of Orthopaedic Surgeons.

Anderson, M., Parr, G., & Hall, S. (2009). *Foundations of athletic training: Prevention assessment, and management* (4th ed.). Philadelphia, PA: Williams & Wilkins.

Bachmann, L., Kolb, E., Koller, M., Steurer, J., & Ter Riet, G.(2003). Accuracy of Ottawa Ankle Rules to Exclude Fractures of the Ankle and Mid-foot: A Systematic Review. *British Medical Journal, 326*(7), 417-419.

Barker, S., Wright, K., & Wright, V. (2001). *Sports injuries 3D* (3rd ed.). Gardner, KS: Cramer Products, Inc.

Hoppenfeld, S. (1976). *Physical examination of the spine and extremities.* New York, NY: Appleton-Century Crofts.

Magee, D. (2002). *Orthopedic physical assessment* (4th ed.). Philadelphia, PA: W.B. Sanders.

Mellion, M., Walsh, W., Madden, C., Putukian, M., & Shelton, G. (2001). The team physician's handbook (3rd ed.). Philadelphia, PA: Hanley and Belfus, Inc.

Neumann, D. (2010). *Kinesiology of the musculoskeletal system: Foundations for rehabilitation* (2nd ed.). St. Louis, MO: Mosby Elsevier.

Perrin, D. (2005). *Athletic taping and bracing* (2nd ed.). Champaign, IL: Human Kinetics.

Pfieffer, R., & Mangus, B. (2011). *Concepts of athletic training* (6th ed.). Boston, MA: Jones and Bartlett.

Prentice, W. (2011). *Arnheim's principles of athletic training: A competency-based approach* (14th ed.). St. Louis, MO: McGraw-Hill Higher Education.

Prentice, W. (2011). *Rehabilitation techniques in sports medicine* (5th ed.). St. Louis, MO: McGraw-Hill Higher Education.

Prentice, W. (2009). *Therapeutic modalities: For sports medicine and athletic training* (6th ed.). St. Louis, MO: McGraw-Hill Higher Education.

Starkey, C., Brown, S., & Ryan, J. (2010). *Examination of orthopedic and athletic injuries* (3rd ed.). Philadelphia, PA: F. A. Davis.

Stedman's medical dictionary for the health professions and nursing (7th ed.). (2011). Baltimore, MD: Williams & Wilkins.

Wright K., Whitehill, W., & Lewis M. (2003). *Preventive techniques: Taping/wrapping techniques and protective devices.* Gardner, KS: Cramer Products.

Wright K., & Whitehill, W. (1996). *The comprehensive manual of taping and wrapping techniques.* Gardner, KS: Cramer Products.

Suggested Multimedia Resources

Wright, K., Harrelson, G., Floyd, R., & Fincher, L. (1995). *Sports medicine evaluation series: The ankle and lower leg.* St. Louis, MO: McGraw-Hill Higher Education.

Wright, K., & Whitehill, W. (1996). *Sports medicine taping series: The ankle, the foot, and lower leg.* St. Louis, MO: McGraw-Hill Higher Education.

Review Questions

Completion

1. The _____ is mounted almost directly on top of the talus and extends over its medial side.

2. The talocrural joint is formed by the _____, _____, and _____.

3. The injured ankle should be compared to the _____ _____.

4. _____ _____ usually refers to a great toe sprain.

5. The four arches of the foot are the _____ _____, _____ _____.

6. Factors that contribute to muscle cramps are: (list 4)

   _____ _____

   _____ _____

7. Two indicators of stress fractures are _____ and _____.

8. The three muscles of the deep posterior compartment are the _____, _____, and the _____ .

9. The large, bony protrusions on each side of the ankle are known as the _____.

10. With inversion ankle sprains, the ligament most often injured is the _____ _____ ligament, on the _____ side of the ankle.

11. A common mechanism of injury for an anterior tibiofibular ligament sprain is _____.

12. When icing an athlete with an ice bag and elastic wrap after an acuteankle sprain, the ice should be applied for at least _____ minutes.

Short Answer

1. Define the acronym:

   H_____ O_____ P_____ S_____

2. Explain the differences between a first, second, and third degree ankle sprain.

3. What is a March fracture?

4. Identify some of the exercises used to rehabilitate the ankle.

5. Define strain to the Achilles tendon.

6. Define a sprain to the great toe.

7. What are the symptoms of anterior compartment syndrome?

8. How are stress fractures evaluated?

9. What is a common complaint with plantar fasciitis?

10. What are the Ottawa Ankle rules?

11. Which muscles are typically strengthened for a patient with medial tibial stress syndrome?

7 Knee and Thigh

Educational Objectives

Upon completing this chapter, the reader will be able to do the following:

- Name the anatomy of the knee and thigh
- Identify the steps in an evaluation format
- Compare the common injuries to the knee and thigh
- Demonstrate the principles of rehabilitation to the knee and thigh
- Describe the preventive/supportive techniques and protective devices for the lower extremity

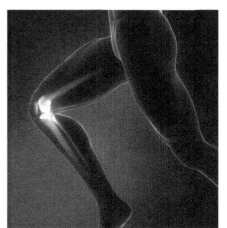

The knee is a complicated joint. When an injury occurs, a thorough evaluation is critical. After the initial first-aid treatment of protection, rest, ice, compression, elevation and support, referral to a physician is recommended. Fortunately, it has been found that many of the more serious knee injuries in sports can be prevented. The key is that the athlete work to strengthen the quadriceps and hamstring muscle groups. For those injuries that do occur, knees that are protected by strong muscles often suffer less severe problems. Rehabilitation time is also reduced if the knee musculature is strong.

Anatomy

The knee is the largest joint in the body. Despite its size, though, it is structurally very weak. The joint's primary weakness is due to its relatively unstable bony structure. To illustrate this instability, consider the femur, or thighbone. The femur is the longest and strongest bone in the body. However, it sits precariously on top of the smaller tibia, which is the main weight-bearing bone of the lower leg. These two bones slide back and forth on each other, even in nonstressful, nonathletic activities. Subtracting further from the joint's stability is the small amount of normal rotation by the femur on the tibia. Not everything in this joint's structure is detrimental to stability. The distal end of the femur has two slightly convex surfaces, called condyles. These condyles articulate with the slightly concave surfaces of the tibia. However, once the knee starts to bend, whether the action is walking, running, or climbing stairs, stability from these convex and concave surfaces is greatly diminished.

The femur and tibia are only two of the four bones of the knee joint. The next largest bone is the fibula, which only bears about 10% of a person's weight. The fibula articulates at the knee only with the tibia, and serves as the attachment for the lateral collateral ligament and biceps femoris muscle. The fourth bone of the knee joint is called the patella, or knee cap. The patella, encased in the powerful patellar tendon, moves up and down in front of the knee in the space between the two condyles of the femur.

The instability of the knee's bony structure is partially compensated for by strong ligaments and potentially even stronger muscle support. Four important ligaments help stabilize the knee: the medial collateral ligament (MCL), the lateral collateral ligament (LCL), the anterior cruciate ligament (ACL), and the posterior cruciate ligament (PCL).

On the medial side of the knee, the broad, flat MCL helps secure the femur to the tibia. This ligament also connects to the cartilage of the knee, the medial meniscus. Located on the lateral side of the knee, the LCL is not quite as strong as the medial ligament. The LCL is a cord-like ligament that does not attach to the lateral meniscus. The collateral ligaments assist in reducing valgus and varus (abduction and adduction of tibia on femur) movement in the knee joint. The two cruciate ligaments form an "x" in the center of the joint (cruciate comes from the Latin word meaning cross). These ligaments control anterior and posterior movement of the femur on the tibia.

More than any other joint, the knee is dependent on good muscle support. In fact, there are 12 muscles that support the anatomical structures of the knee joint. Most of the support comes from the large muscle groups in the thigh and lower leg. The supporting muscle group on the anterior aspect of the thigh is called the quadriceps. The quadriceps group is comprised of: rectus femoris, vastus medialis, vastus lateralis, and vastus intermedius. The quadriceps muscles, which extend (straighten) the lower leg, converge to form the patellar tendon. This tendon encases the patella and inserts on the front of the tibia on the tibial tubercle. The vastus medialis muscle is vital in patellar tracking.

The muscles located on the posterior aspect of the thigh are called the hamstring and include the semitendinosus, semimembranosus, and biceps femoris. The hamstring muscle group flexes (bends) the knee and also helps control the rotary movements of the tibia. Called a natural knee brace by many athletic trainers, the hamstrings originate on the pelvis and femur and divide to attach below the knee on the tibia and fibula. While the quadriceps and hamstrings are most commonly known, other muscles also provide support and control movement of the knee. These muscles include the sartorius, gracilis, popliteus, gastrocnemius, plantaris, and tensor fascia latae/IT band.

The knee joint contains two tough, fibrous cartilages, known as menisci. They are called the lateral meniscus and medial meniscus. These menisci rest on top of the tibia in its two shallow concave indentations. The menisci form a cushioned base for the medial and lateral condyles of the femur. Other functions of the menisci include shock absorption, adding to joint stability and helping to smooth the gliding and rotating movements of the femur and tibia.

Other structures in the knee of special concern in athletics are the bursa, synovial membrane, and fat pads. The bursae are closed, fluid-filled sacs that serve as cushions against friction over a prominent bone, or where a tendon moves over a bone. The synovial membrane is a large, closed sac that lines the inside of the knee joint, helping to lubricate the joint. Fat pads are specialized soft tissue structure for weight bearing and absorbing impact. This area of the body is innervated by a number of different nerves. The sensory distribution of a nerve root is called a dermatome, which produces feeling in a certain anatomical area. The motor distribution of a group of muscles innervated by a single nerve root is called a myotome and it produces movement of the anatomical structures.

Knee, Quadriceps, and Hamstrings Anatomy

Bones
- Femur
- Tibia
- Fibula
- Patella

Ligaments
- Medial collateral (MCL)
- Lateral collateral (LCL)
- Anterior cruciate (ACL)
- Posterior cruciate (PCL)

Cartilage
- Medial meniscus
- Lateral meniscus

Muscles and Tendon and their Functions
- **Vastus medialis:** extension of knee
- **Vastus lateralis:** extension of knee
- **Vastus intermedius:** extension of knee
- **Rectus femoris:** extension of knee, flexion of hip
- **Gracilis:** adduction of hip and flexion of knee
- **Sartorius:** flexion and rotation of hip and knee
- **Semitendinosus:** knee flexion and medial rotation
- **Semimembranosus:** knee flexion and medial rotation
- **Popliteus:** medial rotation and knee flexion
- **Biceps femoris:** flexion of knee and lateral rotation
- **Gastrocnemius:** knee flexion and ankle plantar flexion
- **Plantaris:** knee flexion

To view videos and other materials related to this chapter on the KNEE AND THIGH, see access instructions on the last page of this text.

Dermatomes
- L2—inguinal region: upper two-thirds of anterior thigh (quadriceps) and lateral hamstring
- L3—upper two-thirds of the anterior thigh (quadriceps) and medial hamstring
- L4—anteriomedial aspect of lower leg and rear one-third of foot
- L5—anteriolateral and posterior aspect of lower leg and dorsum of foot
- S1—phalanges and plantar aspect of foot
- S2—proximal one-third of posterior aspect of lower leg

Myotomes
- L2—Hip flexion
- L3—Knee extension
- L4—Dorsiflexion of ankle
- L5—Extensor halluces longus, toe extension
- S1—Plantar flexion of ankle or hamstring curl, foot eversion, hip extension

When determining the strength of myotomes, provide resistive force.

Range of Motion
- Flexion: decreasing angle between the femur and the tibia (e.g., bending the knee)
- Extension: increasing the angle between the femur and the tibia (e.g., straightening the knee)
- Tibial internal rotation: rotation of the tibia toward the midline of the body
- Tibial external rotation: rotation of the tibia away from the midline of the body
- Anterior/posterior translation: movement of the femur on the tibia in a forward (anterior) or backward (posterior) movement pattern

Evaluation Format

The first purpose of an evaluation is to determine if a serious injury has occurred. Initially, a fracture should always be suspected. Signs of a fracture include, but are not limited to, direct or indirect pain, deformity, or a grating sound (i.e., crepitus) at the injury site. Some fractures are not accompanied by swelling or pain. If a fracture is suspected, the extremity should be splinted and the athlete transported for medical evaluation. Young athletes are especially susceptible to fractures, due to their immature bone structure. Often, ligaments and muscles are stronger than the bones. The evaluation process to help determine the type of injury involves four steps: history, observation, palpation, and special tests.

(H) History
This involves asking questions of the athlete to help determine the mechanism of injury. Answers to these questions will help to adequately assess the injury and assist the certified athletic trainer or the physician in a diagnosis.
1. Mechanism of injury (How did it happen?)
2. Location of pain (Where does it hurt?)
3. Sensations experienced (Did you hear a pop or snap?)
4. Previous injury (Have you injured this anatomical structure before?)

(O) Observation
Compare the uninjured to the injured lower extremity and look for bleeding, deformity, swelling, discoloration, scars, and other signs of trauma.

(P) Palpation
Palpation is the physical inspection of an injury. First, palpate the anatomical structures/joints above and below the injuried site. Then palpate the affected area. From knowledge of the lower extremity's anatomy and injury mechanism, the type and extent of injury can be evaluated. Involve the athlete in the evaluation as much as possible. Using bilateral comparison, these items should be palpated/performed:
1. Neurological (motor and sensory)
2. Circulation (pulse and capillary refill)
3. Anatomical Structures (palpate)
4. Fracture test (palpation, compression, and distraction)

(S) Special Tests
With all special tests, the certified athletic trainer is looking for joint instability, disability, and pain. It is possible to further damage an injury through manipulation. These tests are well beyond the expertise of an athletic training student or coach. To determine if damage has been done to the anatomical structures, the certified athletic trainer uses special functional tests to assess disability. These include the following:
1. Joint stability (ligament)
2. Muscle/tendon
3. Accessory anatomical structures
4. Inflammatory conditions
5. Range of motion (active, assistive, passive and resistive)
6. Pain or weakness in the affected area.

Refer to Chapter 2 for a full explanation of the HOPS injury evaluation format.

Conditions that Indicate an Athlete Should Be Referred for Physician Evaluation

- Gross deformity
- Significant pain
- Increased swelling
- Circulation or neurological impairment
- Joint instability
- Dislocated patella
- Abnormal sensations such as clicking, popping, grating, or weakness
- Locked knee or excessively limited motion
- Any doubt regarding the severity or nature of the injury

Common Injuries

The knee joint, due to its complex joint movements, is injured frequently. When an injury occurs, chances of it medical referral and potential surgery is increased. Coaches should not try to determine whether a knee injury is minor or severe. Without advanced medical training, an evaluation is not possible. It is possible for a knee to be severely injured and to exhibit little swelling or pain; therefore, knee injuries call for immediate referral to a physician. In athletics, the most common knee and thigh injuries occur as a result of contusions, sprains, and strains.

Contusions

Contusion injuries are caused by a direct blow or by falling on the knee. A common contusion that can be very painful is the quadriceps contusion. Caused by a direct blow, a quadriceps contusion exhibits moderate to severe pain, spasm, and ecchymosis (discoloration). Due to the spasm of the muscle, producing a knee extension force is severely limited. In addition to ice, compression, and rest, it is recommended to keep the knee flexed as much as possible during the first 24 hours after injury. This knee flexion can reduce the amount of spasm and reduce the amount of swelling that occurs in the area. In some cases, putting the athlete in a knee brace and immobilizing the brace in as much flexion as possible (up to 120 degrees) has shown a quicker return to play. Besides muscular contusions, direct blows or falls can also damage the bursas that protect the bones and other structures of the knee. Since athletes are likely to suffer knee contusions, the basic first-aid treatment is protection, rest, ice, compression, elevation and support. To reduce the occurrence of contusion to the knee itself, kneepads should be worn.

Ligament Sprains

Ligament sprains can be caused by multidirectional forces and are compounded when the athlete's foot is stationary (planted). A common knee sprains occurs in football when a player receives a direct force to the lateral side of the knee joint, called a valgus blow. In this type of injury, the medial ligament is usually stretched and/or torn. The ligaments supporting the knee joint are usually stretched by one of these mechanisms: shearing, torsion, or compression. Torsion injuries occur when the feet are fixed and the body/injured joint is twisted. Shearing occurs when a force is delivered to the opposite side of the joint. Both types of injuries are common. Sports that require cleated shoes pose a greater risk of injury. In fact, the longer the spike is on the cleat, the greater the risk of injury to increased torsion.

A blow severe enough to cause ligament damage will often result in some excessive torsion. Torsion injuries sometimes damage the ligaments, but most often involve the menisci. Other, usually less severe, knee injuries can be caused by muscular weakness or imbalance, overuse, or repetition, poor running mechanics, or improperly fitted shoes. In addition, some athletes are susceptible to certain knee conditions that are related to the growth process.

Whenever the knee joint is evaluated as a sprain, it is usually placed into one of three categories: first degree (mild), second degree (moderate), or third degree (severe).

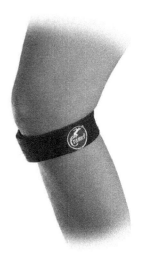

First degree sprain. With a first degree sprain, one or more of the supporting ligaments and surrounding tissues are stretched. There is minor discomfort, point tenderness, and limited or no swelling. There is no abnormal movement in the joint to indicate lack of stability.

Second degree sprain. With this sprain, a portion of one or more ligaments is torn. There is pain, swelling, poin tenderness, and loss of function for several minutes or longer. There is slight abnormal movement in the joint. The athlete may not be able to walk normally and will favor the injured leg.

Third degree sprain. With a third degree sprain, one or more ligaments have been completely torn, resulting in joint instability. There is either extreme pain or little pain (if nerve damage has occurred), loss of function, point tenderness, and rapid swelling. An accompanying fracture is possible.

Meniscus Tears

The menisci are structures made of fibrocartilage that primarily reduce the load placed on the knee and function as "shock absorbers" for the knee. Menisci are usually injured by a torsion (twisting) force while weightbearing. The deepest portion of the MCL also attaches to the medial meniscus, so a second degree or third degree tear of the MCL might also include a tear to the medial meniscus. An "unhappy triad" is when the patient tears their ACL, MCL, and medial meniscus. Unique to the menisci in the knee is the lack of blood flow to the outer one-third of each structure. When an injury occurs to this avascular outer one-third of the menisci, the cartilage is unable to heal on its own and will require surgery to restore complete function to the knee. During a knee surgery (usually an arthroscopy) the physician may perform a partial meniscectomy or a meniscus repair. The partial meniscectomy is when the physician smoothes out the rough edges of the tear, which restores function to the knee. The advantage to this surgery is the speed of returning to play (typically three to six weeks) but also the disadvantage is that there is an increase in the likelihood for the patient developing arthritic changes to the knee in the long term. A meniscus repair occurs when the inner two-thirds of the menisci are injured and the physician can suture the ends of the meniscus together. The blood flow to that portion of the meniscus allows for healing of the structure and less long-term issues in the knee. The disadvantage of the meniscus repair is the length of the rehabiltation and that the patient is typically non-weight bearing (with crutches) for at least 6 weeks.

Patellar Tendinitis

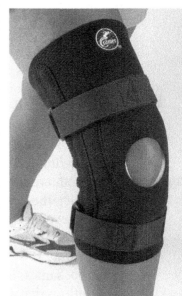

The patellar tendon originates from the quadriceps muscles. The primary action of the quadriceps is knee extension. This movement is part of the jumping process and the forces generated can be great. Excessive stress placed on the patellar tendon can cause inflammation above or below the patella. Pain is reported by the athlete after exercising, in which some swelling may be present. Cold can be utilized to reduce pain and inflammation. The physician may also prescribe rest. As with many knee problems, strong and flexible hamstrings and quadriceps muscles often can prevent or alleviate patellar tendinitis. Additionally, the utilization of eccentric exercises in rehabilitation is helpful.

Chondromalacia Patellae

Chondromalacia patellae is a painful degenerative condition that results in the irritation and softening of the cartilage on the posterior aspect of the patella. Running, jumping, kneeling, and climbing stairs can elicit the pain. One cause of this condition is muscular weakness or imbalance particularly in the hip. This can cause unusual tracking of the patella as it moves in the femoral groove. Other causes of chondromalacia patellae are related to the individual athlete's body structure. Whether the cause is muscular or structural, strengthening the quadriceps through straight leg raises and limited range of motion resistance exercises can often correct the problem. Other treatments include cold application before and after activity, muscle setting (isometric) strengthening exercises, and use of knee pads to protect the area.

The Female Athlete's Knee

Patellar problems may be more prevalent for women than men, because of the structural difference in pelvic girdle width between males and females. The female's wider pelvis creates a sharper angle where the femur attaches to the pelvis. The Q-angle is formed between the line of resultant force produced by the quadriceps, an imaginary line originating from the Anterior Superior Iliac Spine (ASIS) to intersection of an extended line of the patella tendon. A sharper Q-angle changes the line of pull of the quadriceps muscles and may cause the patella to be pulled in a lateral direction upon muscle contraction. Other factor that can increase Q-angle are flat feet and weak hip abductors. Flat feet, pes planus, causes biomechanical changes to the lower extremity and increased rotation of the tibia due to the increased body-weight load on the medial side of the foot. This increased medial force along the medial longitudinal arch, causes an external rotation of the tibia, thereby increasing the patient's Q-angle. A weak hip abductor (gluteus medius) can cause increased hip internal rotation, thus increasing the Q-angle in a patient. This change in mechanics can cause chronic conditions such as chondromalacia patellae, patellar dislocation, or subluxation. If a female athlete is suffering from one of these chronic knee injuries, strengthening the hip abductors, providing support for the medial longitudinal arch, and strengthening the medial portion of the quadriceps (vastus medialis usually prevent any lateral sliding of the patella. Performing complete range of motion exercises with resistance can strengthen the vastus medialis muscle group and the hip abductor group. If chronic knee pain persists, refer the athlete to the team physician. Application of cryotherapy and modification of activity or rest are also recommended.

Osgood-Schlatter Condition

This condition is common to adolescent and is characterized by swelling below one or both knees. It involves the growth center of the tibial tubercle to which the patellar tendon attaches. Depending on its severity, the Osgood-Schlatter condition can lead to chronic knee irritation and pain and was first described early in this century as a partial separation of the tibial tubercle from the tendon. Later, it was described as an inflammation of the tibial tubercle, rather than a bone separation. Regardless of the cause, this inflammation is aggravated by activity and relieved by rest. Tenderness tends to be most marked at the patellar tendon's insertion point. The athlete will complain of severe pain on jumping, running, or kneeling, and after athletic activity. In cases of long duration, the front of the knee appears enlarged and a bony prominence can be felt. Although Osgood-Schlatter symptoms disappear after adolescence, this bony prominence remains. The athlete's physician may recommend treatment ranging from restriction or modification of sports activity to immobilization in a cast.

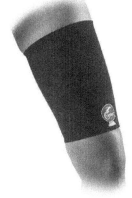

Muscular Strains

Since the quadriceps and hamstrings are located in the thigh, muscular strains are common. Common causes of muscle strains are lack of strength, repetitive overuse, improper technique and inadequate warm-up. When palpating the area, one may note soreness or pain primarily in the soft tissue. Manual resistance to every movement the knee and hip joints can make help reveal the injured muscle. The basic treatment should consist of protection, rest, ice, compression, elevation, and support.

Rehabilitation

Regardless of the mechanism of injury, the typical response to knee injury is basic first aid: protection, rest, ice, compression, elevation, and support, followed by referral to a physician. Muscle strength, power, endurance, and balance is necessary to prevent injury. During strength training, the athlete should work to have the strength of the corresponding muscle group of the injured leg equal to that of the uninjured leg. The best way to build this strength is through resistance exercises or weight training. As with all muscles, strength is lost if the muscle is not exercised regularly. It is therefore important that athletes perform strengthening exercises in-season as well as during the off-season. The sports medicine team should recommend a specific knee rehabilitation program, depending on the injury. Before returning to competition, the following rehabilitation guidelines must be met:

- Full range of motion
- Strength, power, and endurance are proportional to the athlete's size and sport
- No pain during running, jumping, or cutting

Prior to the beginning of any rehabilitation exercise program, the athletic trainer should consult with all members of the sports medicine team and establish an individual program tailored for that individual athlete and the specific injury. The following exercises can be used as rehabilitation exercises or for preventive exercises:

Range of Motion Exercises
- Flexion
- Extension
- Tibial internal rotation
- Tibial external rotation

Knee
- Straight leg raises
- Quadriceps tightening (quad sets)
- Heel slides
- Wall slides
- Step ups
- Leg curls
- Leg extensions

Quadriceps
- Leg extensions
- Straight leg raises
- Hip flexion

Hamstrings
- Leg curls
- Stationary bicycle
- Hip extension

Included in any rehabilitation protocol is the following:
- Range of motion exercises
- Resistive exercises
- Functional activities (walking, squatting, stair climbing, progressive running, cycling)
- Sport-specific activities (jumping, figure of eights, jumping rope, etc.)

Preventive/Supportive Techniques

The application of preventive and supportive techniques is a time-honored and time-consuming tradition. It is also a very expensive practice. Whether to apply adhesive and/or elastic bandages to an uninjured anatomical structure is a decision the athletic trainer will have to make. All injured joints should be supported initially. An outline of basic taping and wrapping techniques for the knee and thigh follows.

Wrapping Techniques for Compression
Knee compression wrap

Wrapping Techniques for Support
Knee joint wrap
Hamstrings wrap
Quadriceps wrap
Hip flexor wrap
Hip adductor wrap

Taping Techniques for the Knee, Thigh, and Hip
Collateral knee
Hyperextended knee
Anterior cruciate
Patella tendon
Hip pointer

Knee Compression Wrap

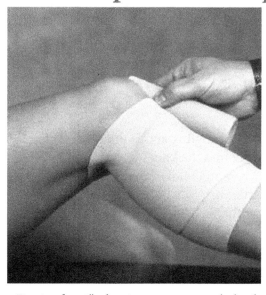 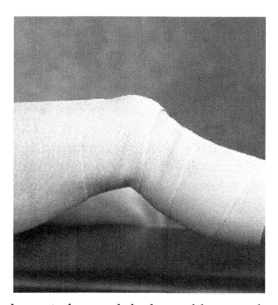

1. Begin the 6" elastic wrap around the lower leg, spiral around the leg and knee, and above the knee.
2. Secure the wrap with a small strip of 1 1/2" adhesive tape.

Knee Joint Wrap

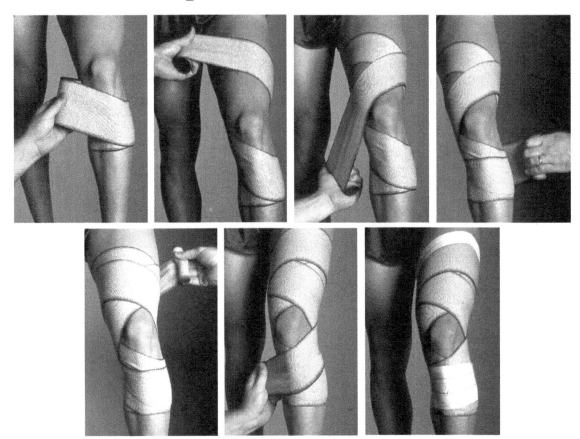

1. Begin the wrap on the lateral/posterior aspect of the lower leg. Encircle the lower leg, moving medially to laterally.
2. Angle the wrap below the patella and cross the medial joint line. Cover the thigh's posterior and lateral aspect.
3. Encircle the thigh, moving medially to laterally. Angle the wrap downward, staying above the patella, and crossing the medial joint line.
4. Cross the popliteal space and encircle the lower leg.
5. Proceed with the wrap, crossing the lateral joint line and angling above the patella.
6. Encircle the thigh and on the posterior aspect, angle across the knee's lateral joint line, staying below the patella. This configuration should resemble a diamond shape around the patella and cover from mid-thigh to the gastrocnemius.
7. Secure this wrap with 1-1/2" adhesive tape, applied at the wrap's loose end.

Hamstring Wrap

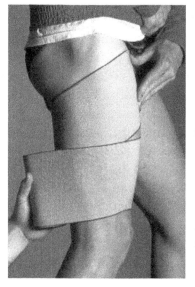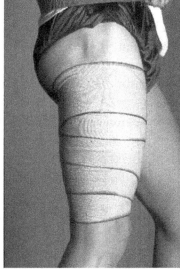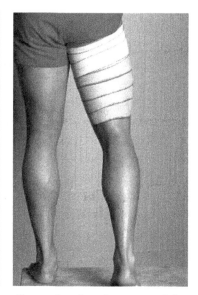

1. Begin the wrap at the thigh's proximal end. Angle diagonally to the distal aspect of the hamstrings. At this point, begin an upward spiral supportive procedure with the wrap. Overlap each layer by one-half its width, ending at the thigh's proximal end.
2. Secure the wrap in place by applying an anchor strip of 1-1/2" adhesive tape.

Quadriceps Wrap

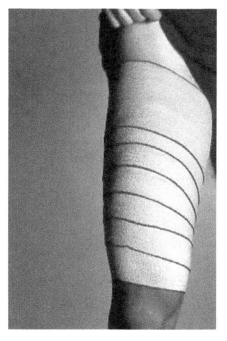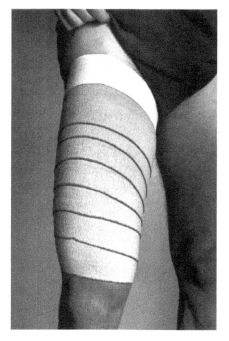

1. Begin the wrap at the thigh's proximal end. Angle diagonally to the distal aspect of the quadriceps. At this point, begin an upward spiral supportive procedure with the wrap. Overlap each layer by one-half its width, ending at the thigh's proximal end.
2. Secure the wrap in place by applying an anchor strip of 1-1/2" adhesive tape.

Preventing ACL Injuries in Female Athletes

Research has found a 4- to 6-fold increase in the number of ACL injuries in women when compared to men (Myer et al., 2004). One of the common mechanisms for injuring the ACL is a non-contact mechanism, where the athlete goes to plant the foot and turn directions, causing a torsion of the ACL and a rupture of the ligament. There have been many theories of why this occurs in women more than man with some research pointing to a difference in neuromuscular control during landing and jumping activities. Research has found that women tend to land from a jump in a more straight-legged position than men and tend to rely on the ligaments to give stability to the knee, whereas men tend to land with more of a bent knee and rely on the musculature of the leg to give stability to the knee. Several different ACL prevention programs has been developed recently to try to decrease the incidence of ACL injuries, specifically non-contact ACL tears. Many ACL prevention programs for females focus on strengthening the hamstring muscle group, plyometrics and agility drills, all while focusing on proper biomechanical techniques such as landing on the toes with the knee bending over the foot instead of in a valgus position. The study by Mandlebaum (2005), found an 88% decrease in ACL injuries amongst high-school aged female soccer players who participated in a specific ACL prevention program.

Protective Devices

The use of protective devices is beneficial if they are properly selected, used in the appropriate setting, correctly fitted, properly applied, and used within the rules and guidelines of the specific sport. Consultation with an equipment specialist and certified athletic trainer is highly encouraged. Listed below are various protective devices that are commercially available to use as an adjunct or replacement to a taping or wrapping procedures.

- Closed/open patella neoprene sleeve
- Hinged knee brace
- Knee brace
- Knee wraps for weight lifting
- Lateral patella subluxation braces
- Osgood-Schlatter condition braces
- Patella stabilizing strap
- Patella tendon tendinitis braces
- Patella tendon strap
- Pre-patella bursitis protectors
- Prophylactics knee brace: Rehabilitative and functional
- Sport-specific pads (football, volleyball, basketball, wrestling)

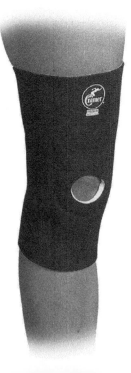
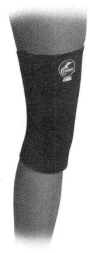
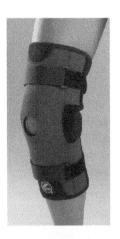

Musculoskeletal Conditions/Disorders

Listed below are conditions/disorders that affect the knee, quadriceps, and/or hamstrings. Using a medical dictionary, review and define these conditions/disorders:
- Bursitis (suprapatella, infrapatella, etc.)
- Dislocation (patella, knee)
- Fracture (patella, tibia, fibula)
- Iliotibial band friction syndrome
- Meniscal tear
- Myositis ossificans
- Osteochondritis dissecans
- Popliteal cyst

References

American Academy of Orthopaedic Surgeons. (2000). *Athletic training and sports medicine.* Chicago, IL: American Academy of Orthopaedic Surgeons.

Anderson, M., Parr, G., & Hall, S. (2009). *Foundations of athletic training: Prevention assessment and management* (4th ed.). Philadelphia, PA: Williams & Wilkins.

Bachmann, L., Kolb, E., Koller, M., Steurer, J., & Ter Riet, G. (2003). Accuracy of Ottawa Ankle Rules to Exclude Fractures of the Ankle and Mid-foot: A Systematic Review. *British Medical Journal, 326*(7), 417-419.

Barker, S., Wright, K., & Wright, V. (2001). *Sports injuries 3D* (3rd ed.). Gardner, KS: Cramer Products, Inc.

Hoppenfeld, S. (1976). *Physical examination of the spine and extremities.* New York, NY: Appleton-Century Crofts.

Magee, D. (2002). *Orthopedic physical assessment* (4th ed.). Philadelphia, PA: W. B. Sanders.

Mandelbaum, B., Silvers, H., Watanabe, D., Knarr, J., Thomas, S., Griffin, L., Kirkendall, D., & Garrett Jr., W. (2005). Effectiveness of a Neuromuscular and Proprioceptive Training Program in Preventing Anterior Cruciate Ligament Injuries in Female Athletes. *American Journal of Sports Medicine, 33*(7), 1003-1010.

Mellion, M., Walsh, W., Madden, C., Putukian, M., & Shelton, G. (2001). *The team physician's handbook* (3rd ed.). Philadelphia, PA: Hanley and Belfus, Inc.

Myer, G., Ford, K., & Hewett, T. (2004). Rationale and Clinical Techniques for Anterior Cruciate Ligament Injury Prevention Among Female Athletes. *Journal of Athletic Training, 39*(4), 352-364.

Neumann, D. (2010). *Kinesiology of the musculoskeletal system: Foundations for rehabilitation* (2nd ed.). St. Louis, MO: Mosby Elsevier.

Perrin, D. (2005). *Athletic taping and bracing* (2nd ed.). Champaign, IL: Human Kinetics.

Pfieffer, R., & Mangus, B. (2011). *Concepts of athletic training* (6th ed.). Boston, MA: Jones and Bartlett.

Prentice, W. (2011). *Arnheim's principles of athletic training: A competency-based approach* (14th ed.). St. Louis, MO: McGraw-Hill Higher Education.

Prentice, W. (2011). *Rehabilitation techniques in sports medicine* (5th ed.). St. Louis, MO: McGraw-Hill Higher Education.

Prentice, W. (2009). *Therapeutic modalities: For sports medicine and athletic training* (6th ed.). St. Louis, MO: McGraw-Hill Higher Education.

Starkey, C., Brown, S., & Ryan, J. (2010). *Examination of orthopedic and athletic injuries* (3rd ed.). Philadelphia, PA: F. A. Davis.

Stedman's medical dictionary for the health professions and nursing (7th ed.). (2011). Baltimore, MD: Williams & Wilkins.

Wright, K., Whitehill, W., & Lewis, M. (2003). *Preventive techniques: Taping/wrapping techniques and protective devices.* Gardner, KS: Cramer Products.

Wright, K., & Whitehill, W. (1996). *The comprehensive manual of taping and wrapping techniques.* Gardner, KS: Cramer Products.

Suggested Multimedia Resources

Wright, K., Harrelson, G., Floyd, R., & Fincher, L. (1995). *Sports medicine evaluation series: The knee.* St. Louis, MO: McGraw-Hill Higher Education.

Wright, K., & Whitehill, W. (1996). *Sports medicine taping series: The knee.* St. Louis, MO: McGraw-Hill Higher Education.

Review Questions

Completion

1. While the knee is the largest joint in the body; structurally it is very _____.

2. The main weight bearing bone of the lower leg is the _____.

3. The slightly concave surfaces of the distal tibia are called the _____.

4. The _____ ligaments assist in reducing valgus and varus (abduction and adduction of tibia on femur) movement in the knee, while the _____ ligaments control anterior and posterior movement of the femur on the tibia.

5. The four muscles that comprise the quadriceps group are the _____, _____, _____, and _____.

6. _____ _____ condition is related to the growth center at the tibial tubercle.

Short Answer

1. How does a torsion injury occur to the knee joint?

2. What structures are injured in an "unhappy triad"?

3. What are the functions of the menisci?

4. Describe the Osgood-Schlatter condition. Why is it common to adolescents?

5. What are some common causes of hamstring and quadriceps muscle strains?

6. Give three biomechanical reasons why patellar problems might occur.

7. What criteria would be used to determine when the athlete is ready to return to sports participation?

8. Name the four most important ligaments of the knee.

9. What condition is characterized by an irritation and softening of the cartilage on the posterior aspect of the patella?

10. Why might females be more likely to tear their ACL than males? How would you prevent this injury?

8 Hip and Pelvis

Educational Objectives

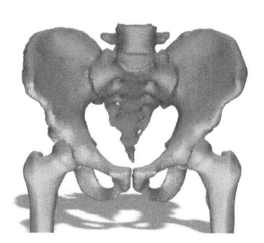

The learner should, at the completion of the chapter, be able to perform the following:
- Name the anatomy of the hip and pelvis
- Identify the components of an injury evaluation format
- Compare the common injuries associated with the hip and pelvis
- Demonstrate the protocol for a rehabilitation program to the hip and pelvis
- Describe the preventive/supportive techniques and protective devices for the hip and pelvis

Anatomy

The arrangement of bones, ligaments, muscles, and tendons make the hip the strongest joint in the body. The hip joint is a ball and socket joint. It is formed by the spherical head of the femur fitting into the deep socket of the hip. There are three bones of the pelvis: the ilium, ischium, and pubis. Attached to the pelvis are groin and torso muscles that are involved in supporting and moving the trunk and upper and lower extremities. These hip and pelvis bones are supported by these ligaments: ligamentum teres, transverse acetabular, iliofemoral, pubofemoral, and inguinal. The bones of the hip and pelvic region provide the structure to transfer weight between the torso and the lower extremities.

There are a number of important muscle groups that are located at the hip and pelvic region. The largest muscle group includes the gluteal muscles. The gluteus maximus, gluteus medius, and gluteus minimus assist in hip extension, abduction, and internal and external rotation (respectively). Muscles that assist in hip flexion are the iliopsoas, sartorius, pectineus, and rectus femoris. Hip adduction is performed by the group of muscles known as the adductors. The hip adductor group is composed of the adductor longus, adductor brevis, and adductor magnus. The muscle groups that compose the bulk of the thigh (quadriceps and hamstrings) also assist in the movement of the hip. Those movements are hip flexion and hip extension, respectively.

This area of the body is innervated by a number of different nerves. The sensory distribution of a nerve root is called a dermatome, which produces feeling in a certain anatomical area. The motor distribution of a group of muscles innervated by a single nerve root is called a mytome, and it produces movement of anatomical structures. Additional anatomical structures frequently injured are fat pads and bursi. Fat pads are specialized soft tissue structures for weight bearing and absorbing impact, whereas synovial sac generally located over bony prominences throughout the body are called bursae.

Hip and Pelvis Anatomy

Bones
Femur
Pelvis (ilium, ischium, pubis)
Sacrum (five fused vertebrae)
Coccyx (four fused vertebrae)

Ligaments—Hip
Ligamentum teres
Transverse acetabular ligament
Iliofemoral ligament
Pubofemoral ligament
Inguinal
Sacroiliac

To view videos and other materials related to this chapter on the HIP AND PELVIS, see access instructions on the last page of this text.

Muscles and Functions
Gluteus maximus: extension of hip
Gluteus medius: abduction and rotation of hip
Gluteus minimus: abduction and rotation of hip
Tensor fascia latae: flexion and internal rotation of hip
Iliacus: flexion of hip
Psoas major: flexes hip, flexes vertebral column
Sartorius: flexion and rotation of hip and knee
Pectineus: adduction and flexion of hip
Adductor longus: adduction and flexion of hip
Adductor brevis: adduction and flexion of hip
Adductor magnus: adduction and flexion of hip
Gracilis: adduction of hip and flexion of knee
Piriformis: lateral rotator
Obturator internus/externus: lateral rotator
Gamellus superior/inferior: lateral rotator
Quadratus femoris: lateral rotator
Biceps femoris: flexion of knee and lateral rotation of leg
Semimembranosus: flexion of the knee, medial rotation of leg
Semitendinosus: flexion of the knee, medial rotation of the leg
Rectus femoris: extension of knee, flexion of hip
Vastus medialis: extension of knee
Vastus lateralis: extension of knee
Vastus intermedius: extension of knee

Anatomical Planes
Sagittal plane: bisecting body into right and left halves
Frontal plane: bisecting the body into front and back halves
Transverse plane: bisecting body into upper and lower halves

Range of Motion—HIP
Adduction: moving leg toward midline in frontal plane
Abduction: moving leg away from midline of body in frontal plane

Pelvic girdle

the bony ring that is composed of the two innominate bones, the sacrum, and the coccyx

Quadriceps

Rectus femoris
Vastus lateralis
Vastus medialis
Vastus intermedius

Hamstrings

Biceps femoris
Semitendinosus
Semimembranosus

"Groin muscles"

Pectineus
Adductor Longus
Adductor Brevis
Adductor Magnus
Gracilis

Flexion: decreasing angle between anterior thigh and abdomen through the sagittal plane
Extension: increasing angle between anterior thigh and abdomen through the sagittal plane
Internal rotation: rotation of femur toward midline
External rotation: rotation of femur away from midline

Range of Motion—TORSO

Flexion: moving the torso forward through the sagittal plane
Extension: moving the torso backward through the sagittal plane
Lateral flexion: moving the torso laterally (side to side) in the frontal plane
Rotation: rotating the torso in the transverse plane

Dermatones

L1—inguinal region
L2—inguinal region and upper two-thirds of anterior thigh (quadriceps) and lateral hamstring
L3—upper two-thirds of the anterior thigh (quadriceps) and medial hamstring
L4—anteriomedial aspect of lower leg and rear one-third of foot
L5—anteriolateral and posterior aspect of lower leg and dorsum of foot
S1—phalanges and plantar aspect of foot
S2—proximal one-third of posterior aspect of lower leg

Myotomes

L2—Hip flexion
L3—Knee extension
L4—Dorsiflexion of ankle
L5—Extensor halluces longus, toe extension
S1—Plantar flexion of ankle or hamstring curl, foot eversion, hip extension
S2—Dorsiflexion of foot

When determining the strength of myotomes, provide resistive force.

Dermatome

a segment of the skin that is innervated by a spinal nerve

Innervated

nerve stimulation (usually of a muscle)

Evaluation Format

The first purpose of an evaluation is to determine if a serious injury has occurred. Initially, a fracture should always be suspected. Signs of a fracture include, but are not limited to, direct or indirect pain, deformity, or a grating sound at the injury site. Some fractures are not accompanied by swelling or pain. If a fracture is suspected, the extremity should be splinted and emergency medical services (EMS) should be notified to transport the injured athlete. Young athletes are especially susceptible to fractures, due to their immature bone structure. Often, ligaments and muscles are stronger than the bones. The evaluation process to help determine the type of injury involves four steps: history, observation, palpation, and special tests.

(H) History

This involves asking questions of the athlete to help determine the mechanism of injury. Answers to these questions will help to adequately assess the injury and assist the certified athletic trainer or the physician in a diagnosis:
1. Mechanism of injury (How did it happen?)
2. Location of pain (Where does it hurt?)
3. Sensations experienced (Did you hear a pop or snap?)
4. Previous injury (Have you injured this anatomical structure before?)

(O) Observation

Compare the uninjured to the injured lower extremity and look for bleeding, deformity, swelling, discoloration, scars, and other signs of trauma.

(P) Palpation

Palpation is the physical inspection of an injury. First, palpate the anatomical structures/joints above and below the injuried site. Then, palpate the affected area. From knowledge of the lower extremity's anatomy and injury mechanism, the type and extent of injury can be evaluated. Involve the athlete in the evaluation as much as possible. Using bilateral comparison, these items should be palpated/performed:

1. Neurological (motor and sensory)
2. Circulation (pulse and capillary refill)
3. Anatomical structures (palpate)
4. Fracture test (palpation, compression, and distraction)

(S) Special Tests

With all special tests, the certified athletic trainer is looking for joint instability, disability, and pain. It is possible to further damage an injury through manipulation. These tests are well beyond the expertise of an athletic training student or coach. To determine if damage has been done to the anatomical structures, the certified athletic trainer uses special functional tests to assess disability. These include the following:

1. Joint stability (ligament)
2. Muscle/tendon
3. Accessory anatomical structures
4. Inflammatory conditions
5. Range of motion (active, assistive, passive, and resistive)
6. Pain or weakness in the affected area

Refer to Chapter 2 for a full explanation of the HOPS injury evaluation format.

Conditions that Indicate an Athlete Should Be Referred for Physician Evaluation

- Gross deformity
- Significant pain
- Increased swelling
- Circulation or neurological impairment
- Joint instability
- Suspected fracture or dislocation
- Persistent pain in hip and pelvis area
- Noticeable and palpable deficit in the muscle or tendon
- Abnormal sensations such as clicking, popping, grating, or weakness
- Any doubt regarding the severity or nature of the injury

Common Injuries

Injury to the Coccyx

The four fused vertebrae on the lower end of the spine are called the coccyx, or tailbone. Often, this area is bruised from falling on a hard surface. Most injuries to the coccyx will be contusions, although severe trauma could cause a dislocation or fracture. Contusions are treated with the basic treatment of protection, rest, ice, and use of foam padding for sitting or activity.

Hip Strains

Hip strains commonly occur when the joint has received violent twisting motions of the torso accompanied by the feet being fixed in a stationary position. When evaluating hip strains, have the athlete perform various range of movement (flexion, extension, adduction, adduction, circumduction) exercises. Application of basic treatment and use of compression girdles or elastics wrap will aid in support. If chronic pain exists referral to a physician is recommended.

Trochanteric Bursitis

Trochanteric bursitis occurs at the bursae sac at the gluteus medius/iliotibial band insertion at greater trochanter. Running technique should be examined as well as running on level and soft surfaces. If the condition is chronic, the application of heat to the area will help to reduce the chronic irritation.

Trauma to the Genitalia

Injuries to the male genitalia are common, resulting from a direct blow or testicular torsion, which causes excruciating pain and temporary disability. A contusion to the testes will produce the same physiological tissue reaction as contusions to other body parts. There is hemorrhaging, fluid effusion, and muscle spasm. Although less common, female athletes can suffer trauma to the reproductive system. One method to relieve this spasm is to have the athlete lie on the ground and to flex their thighs to their chest. Additionally, have the athlete loosen the clothing area. First-aid treatment should include reducing the spasm, applying a cold pack to the affected area, and referral to a physician for medical evaluation.

Hip Pointer

Some of the muscles that control trunk movement attach to the iliac crest. Due to limited natural protection, injuries to the iliac crest result from direct blow, (contusion) and can disable an athlete. If the force is severe, the muscles that attach at the crest of the ilium are bruised and the injury is called a hip pointer. With all hip pointers, there is immediate pain and swelling may or may not be present. Any movement requiring involvement of the trunk and extremities will result in more pain and discomfort. Extreme caution should be taken when treating this injury. Basic treatment of protection, rest, ice, compression, support, and medical re-evaluation should be incorporated.

Hip Dislocation

While not common, a hip dislocation is a dangerous condition that should only be handled by emergency medical personnel. In most cases, the athlete will be lying on his or her back with the injured extremity flexed and externally rotated. These injuries are usually caused by abnormal stress and the joint will be dislocated either anteriorly or posteriorly. Never attempt to reduce such a dislocation. Nerves and blood vessels could become permanently damaged by the head of the femur. An athlete who has suffered this suspected injury must be handled and transported by qualified medical personnel.

Osteitis Pubis

According to Lynch and Renstrom (1999), osteitis pubis is inflammation and pain at the pubic symphysis of the pelvis which can refer pain to the hip, groin, lower abdomen, and genitalia area. It is thought that stiffness and restricted motion of the hip joint may cause an increase in movement (over 2mm) at the pubic symphysis. Men seem to be affected more than women and more often in soccer players and runners. Fortunately, it appears that one of the best treatments for this condition is to decrease the amount of activity (especially jumping activities or activities involving the groin muscles) of the athlete for about six to nine months and then gradually return to previous levels of competition.

Youth Hip Injuries

Two hip injuries are of particular concern to those involved with youth sports. A Slipped Capital Femoral Epiphysis (SCFE) is an injury to the growth plate of the head of the femur and is most likely to occur in boys aged 10 to 14. In a SCFE, the growth plate slides anteriorly while the head of the femur remains aligned with the acetabulum within the joint. This movement of the epiphysis results in a painful walk with toe-out gait with the athlete complaining of pain when moving the hip into internal rotation. In addition, in nearly 50% of the adolescent patients that develop SCFE, they will also develop an avascular necrosis (death of tissue due to lack of blood) of the femoral head. This avascular necrosis will most likely lead to surgery at some point and delay, if not permanently discontinue, an adolescent's athletic career. Similarly, another hip injury that is more likely in boys than girls and is painful in hip internal rotation is Legg-Calve-Perthes Disease, an avascular necrosis of the femoral head and most often seen in boys prior to the age of 10. Due to the avascular necrosis the femoral head appears in a more flat-like shape rather than a rounder convex shape and will cause a loss of abduction and internal rotation of the hip and will also predispose the young athlete to more arthritis of the hip in later years.

Rehabilitation

Sending an athlete back to competition before healing is complete leaves the player susceptible to further injury. The best way to determine when healing is complete is by the absence of pain during stressful activity and by the return of pain free full range of motion and strength. Before returning to competition, the following rehabilitation guidelines must be met:
- Full range of motion
- Strength, power, and endurance are proportional to the athlete's size and sport
- No pain during running, jumping, or cutting

Prior to the beginning of any rehabilitation exercise program, the athletic trainer should consult with all members of the sports medicine team and establish an individual program tailored for that individual athlete and the specific injury. The following exercises can be used as rehabilitation exercises or for preventive exercises:

Range of Motion Exercises
Hip
    Adduction
    Abduction
    Flexion
    Extension
    Internal rotation
    External rotation
    Circumduction
    Torso flexion
    Extension
    Lateral flexion
    Rotation

Resistance/Strengthening Exercises: Hip and Pelvis
    Abdominal sit-up/curl-ups
    Abdominal crunches

Pelvic tilts
Squats

Included in any rehabilitation protocol are the following:

- Range-of-motion exercises
- Resistance exercises
- Cardiovascular/fitness activities (walking, stair climbing, running, swimming, cycling, etc)
- Sport-specific activities (jumping, figure of eights, cutting, jumping rope, etc.)

Preventive/Supportive Techniques

An outline of basic taping and wrapping techniques utilized to support the hip and pelvis is listed below.

Wrapping Techniques for Support
Hamstrings wrap
Quadriceps wrap
Hip flexor wrap
Hip adductor wrap

Taping Techniques for the Hip and Pelvic
Hip pointer
Low back
Rib

Protective Devices

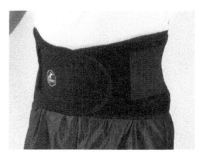

An outline of potential protectives devices that can be utilized to protect the hip and pelvis is listed below. The use of protective devices is beneficial. Consultation with an equipment specialist and certified athletic trainer is highly encouraged.

- Athletic supporter with cup
- Back brace
- Breast support bra
- Low back brace/support
- Rib protector
- Thigh sleeve
- Shoulder pads
- Sport-specific pads
- Sports compression girdle
- Sternum protector

Hip Flexor Wrap

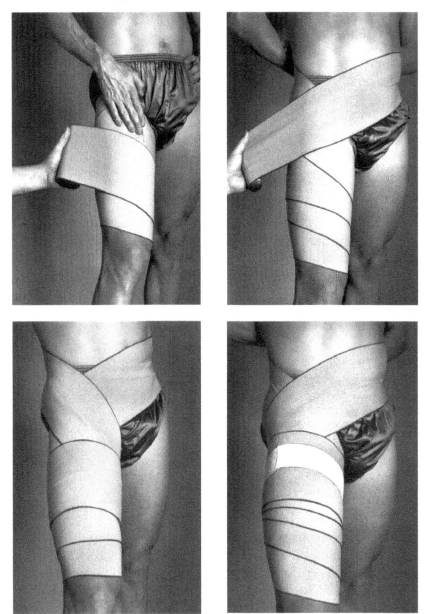

1. Begin the wrap at the proximal end of the thigh. From the anterior surface, angle diagonally to the distal lateral aspect of the quadriceps. Above the knee, begin an upward spiral supportive procedure with the wrap. Overlap each layer by one-half its width.
2. At the proximal end of the thigh, continue the wrap around the waist, pulling to the lateral and posterior aspect.
3. Once the waist has been encircled, continue the wrap around the thigh two to three times.
4. At this point, continue the wrap around the waist. This upward and outward pull should assist in hip flexion and limit hip extension. End the wrap on the thigh. Secure the wrap in place by applying an anchor strip of 1-1/2" adhesive tape.

Hip Adductor Wrap

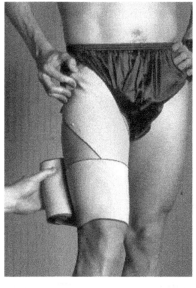
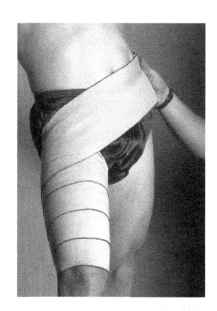
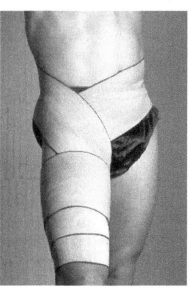
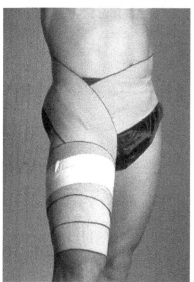

1. Begin the wrap at the proximal end of the thigh. From the anterior surface, angle diagonally to the distal medial aspect of the quadriceps. Above the knee, begin an upward spiral supportive procedure with the wrap. Overlap each layer by one-half its width.
2. At the proximal end of the thigh, continue the wrap around the waist, pull across the abdomen, to the lateral aspect, and then to the posterior aspect. This upward and anterior pull should assist in hip adduction and limit hip abduction.
3. Once the waist has been encircled, continue the wrap downward and around the quadriceps muscle group two to three times.
4. At this point, pull the wrap around the waist, crossing the abdomen, lateral, and posterior aspects. End the wrap on the thigh. Secure the wrap in place by applying an anchor strip of 1-1/2" adhesive tape.

Musculoskeletal Conditions/Disorders

Listed below are musculoskeletal conditions/disorders that affect the hip and pelvis. A valuable learning experience would be to define and review these conditions using a medical dictionary.

- Contusion of the thigh
- Fracture (pelvis or femur)
- Snapping hip syndrome
- Iliotibial band friction syndrome
- Sports hernia
- Piriformis syndrome
- Sprain
- Tendinitis

References

American Academy of Orthopaedic Surgeons. (2000). *Athletic training and sports medicine.* Chicago, IL: American Academy of Orthopaedic Surgeons.

Anderson, M., Parr, G., & Hall, S. (2009). *Foundations of athletic training: Prevention, assessment, and management* (4th ed.). Philadelphia, PA: Williams & Wilkins.

Bachmann, L., Kolb, E., Koller, M., Steurer, J., & Ter Riet, G. (2003). Accuracy of Ottawa Ankle Rules to Exclude Fractures of the Ankle and Mid-foot: A Systematic Review. *British Medical Journal, 326*(7), 417-419.

Barker, S., Wright, K., & Wright, V. (2001). *Sports injuries 3D* (3rd ed.). Gardner, KS: Cramer Products, Inc.

Hoppenfeld, S. (1976). *Physical examination of the spine and extremities.* New York, NY: Appleton-Century Crofts.

Lynch, S., & Renstrom, P. (1999). Groin injuries in sport: Treatment strategies. *Sports Medicine, 28*(2), 137-144.

Magee, D. (2002). *Orthopedic physical assessment* (4th ed.). Philadelphia, PA: W. B. Sanders.

Mandelbaum, B., Silvers, H., Watanabe, D., Knarr, J., Thomas, S., Griffin, L., Kirkendall, D., & Garrett Jr., W. (2005). Effectiveness of a Neuromuscular and Proprioceptive Training Program in Preventing Anterior Cruciate Ligament Injuries in Female Athletes. *American Journal of Sports Medicine, 33*(7), 1003-1010.

Mellion, M., Walsh, W., Madden, C., Putukian, M., & Shelton, G. (2001). *The team physician's handbook* (3rd ed.). Philadelphia, PA: Hanley and Belfus, Inc.

Myer, G., Ford, K., & Hewett, T. (2004). Rationale and Clinical Techniques for Anterior Cruciate Ligament Injury Prevention Among Female Athletes. *Journal of Athletic Training, 39*(4), 352-364.

Neumann, D. (2010). *Kinesiology of the musculoskeletal system: Foundations for rehabilitation* (2nd ed.). St. Louis, MO: Mosby Elsevier.

Perrin, D. (2005). *Athletic taping and bracing* (2nd ed.). Champaign, IL: Human Kinetics.

Pfieffer, R., & Mangus, B. (2011). *Concepts of athletic training* (6th ed.). Boston, MA: Jones and Bartlett.

Prentice, W. (2011). *Arnheim's principles of athletic training: A competency-based approach* (14th ed.). St. Louis, MO: McGraw-Hill Higher Education.

Prentice, W. (2011). *Rehabilitation techniques in sports medicine* (5th ed.). St. Louis, MO: McGraw-Hill Higher Education.

Prentice, W. (2009). *Therapeutic modalities: For sports medicine and athletic training* (6th ed.). St. Louis, MO: McGraw-Hill Higher Education.

Starkey, C., Brown, S., & Ryan, J. (2010). *Examination of orthopedic and athletic injuries* (3rd ed.). Philadelphia, PA: F. A. Davis.

Stedman's medical dictionary for the health professions and nursing (7th ed.). (2011). Baltimore, MD: Williams & Wilkins.

Wright, K., Whitehill W., & Lewis M. (2003). *Preventive techniques: Taping/wrapping techniques and protective devices.* Gardner, KS: Cramer Products.

Wright, K., & Whitehill, W. (1996). *The comprehensive manual of taping and wrapping techniques.* Gardner, KS: Cramer Products.

Suggested Multimedia Resources

Wright, K., Harrelson, G., Floyd, R., & Fincher, L. (1995). *Sports medicine evaluation series: The knee.* St. Louis, MO: McGraw-Hill Higher Education.

Wright, K., & Whitehill, W. (1996). *Sports medicine taping series: The knee.* St. Louis, MO: McGraw-Hill Higher Education.

Review Questions

Completion

1. The hip joint is formed by the spherical head of the _____ fitting into the deep _____ of the hip.
3. The _____ joint is the strongest in the body.

Short Answer

1. What type of joint is the hip?

2. What injury occurs to the growth plate of the head of the femur and is most likely to occur in boys aged 10 to 14?

3. What injury is an avascular necrosis of the femoral head and most often seen in boys prior to the age of 10?

4. What is thought as the primary cause of osteitis pubis?

5. In a hip dislocation, what is the typical position of the hip?

6. What are methods to decrease the spasm caused by trauma to the genitalia?

7. What movements will increase pain during a severe iliac crest contusion?

8. What is the definition of "avascular necrosis"?

9. What rehabilitation exercises may be done to return an athlete who has suffered a thigh or hip injury back to full sports participation?

10. What hip muscles primarily work to abduct and rotate the hip?

9 Thorax and Abdomen

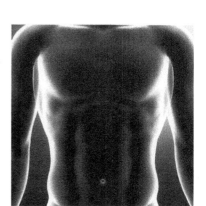

The thorax, better known as the chest cavity, is the area that contains the heart, lungs, esophagus, and the "great vessels," which are the aorta and two venae cavae. The second major body cavity is the abdomen, which contains the major organs for both digestion and excretion.

Educational Objectives

Upon completing this chapter, the reader will be able to do the following:
- Recognize and identify anatomical structures of the thorax and abdomen
- Express the importance of the primary survey
- Express the importance of the secondary survey
- Identify musculoskeletal conditions/disorders of the thorax and abdomen
- Recognize special tests used to evaluate injuries of the thorax and abdomen
- Describe the rehabilitation protocol for the thorax and abdomen
- Recognize preventative/supportive techniques for the thorax and abdomen
- Differentiate protective devices for the thorax and abdomen

Anatomy of the Thorax and Abdomen

Thoracic Compartments
- Right chest (right lung and pulmonary vessels)
- Left chest (left lung and pulmonary vessels)
- Mediastinum (heart, pericardial sac, great vessels, trachea, esophagus)

Abdominal Compartments
- Peritoneal cavity (most solid and hollow organs)
- Retroperitoneal cavity (great vessels, kidneys, and portions of colon)

The above compartments are separated by the diaphragm.

Bones Surrounding the Above Compartments
Thoracic
- Sternum (anteriorly)
- Thoracic vertebrae (12 posteriorly)
- Abdominal
- Lumbar vertebrae (5 posteriorly)

- Sacral vertebrae (5 posteriorly)
- Coccygeal vertebrae (4 fused posteriorly)
- Pelvis (inferiorly)

Muscles of the Thorax and Abdomen and Their Functions
- Pectoralis major (pulls rib cage up, adducts arm, rotates arm medially, primary arm flexor
- Pectoralis minor (draws scapula anteriorly and inferiorly, draws rib cage superiorly)
- Latissimus dorsi (extends upper arm, adducts upper arm posteriorly)
- External intercostals (lifts the rib cage)
- Rectus abdominus (flexes and rotates lumbar region)
- Internal abdominis oblique (aids rectus abdominus, aids the back muscles in trunk rotation and lateral flexion)
- External abdominis oblique (aids rectus abdominus, aids the back muscles in trunk rotation and lateral flexion)
- Transversus abdominis (compresses abdominal contents)

Anatomical Planes
- Sagittal plane (bisects the body into right and left halves)
- Transverse plane (bisects the body into upper and lower halves)
- Frontal plane (bisects the body into front and back halves)

Internal Organs of Thorax
- The heart is located in the central third of the thoracic cavity (mediastinum) and extends slightly to the left. Its function is to pump oxygenated blood to itself and other organs of the body while pumping deoxygenated blood back to the lungs for reoxygenation.
- The lungs are located in the left and right thorax and are protected by the rib cage. They are made up by a network of branching tubes and air sacs that are responsible for oxygen extraction and CO_2 expulsion.
- The great vessels carry blood to and from the heart and lungs.
- The trachea allows for gas exchange between lungs and the air.
- The esophagus carries food from mouth to stomach.

Internal Organs of Abdomen (Divided into four quadrants)
Right Upper
- Liver, gallbladder, pylorus of stomach, head of pancreas, hepatic flexure of colon, portion of small intestine, right kidney, and adrenal gland

Left Upper
- Stomach, spleen, body and tail of pancreas, splenic flexure of colon, portion of small intestine, left kidney, and adrenal gland

Right Lower
- Appendix, cecum of colon, portion of small bowel, right side of urinary, and reproductive system

Left Lower
- Sigmoid colon, rectum, portion of small bowel, left side of urinary, and reproductive system

Hollow Organs of Abdomen
- Stomach
- Small bowel

- Colon
- Gallbladder
- Urinary bladder
- Great vessels

Solid Organs of Abdomen
- Spleen
- Liver
- Kidneys
- Pancreas
- Reproductive organs

Musculoskeletal Disorders or Conditions

Listed below are a number of disorders or conditions that affect the thorax and abdomen. Using a medical dictionary, define/review the following:

Thorax
- arrhythmia
- bradycardia
- tachycardia
- costochondral sprains/separations/contusion
- muscular strain
- rupture of pectoralis major
- rib contusion
- pulmonary contusion
- sternal fracture
- sternoclavicular dislocation
- spontaneous pneumothorax
- traumatic pneumothorax
- tension pneumothorax
- hemothorax
- hemopneumothorax
- flail chest

Abdomen
- dysphagia
- dysmenorrhea
- gastroenteritis
- muscular strain
- hernia
- hematoma/contusion
- pneumoperitoneum
- hemoperitoneum
- peritonitis
- ileus

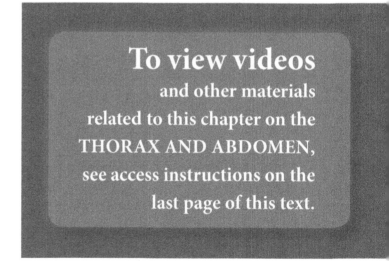

To view videos and other materials related to this chapter on the THORAX AND ABDOMEN, see access instructions on the last page of this text.

Evaluation of the Thorax and Abdomen

Thoracic and abdominal injuries are less common than extremity injuries. However, these injuries can potentially be more life threatening. In order to provide appropriate care, these injuries demand immediate evaluation and, if indicated, subsequent activation of the emergency medical system (EMS).

This chapter outlines general evaluation procedures used to assess thoracic and abdominal injuries. A slight deviation from the HOPS injury evaluation format is presented. Specifically, your evaluation must follow a precise assessment process including a primary then secondary survey. With a basic knowledge of the anatomical components of the thorax and abdomen, their functions and specific conditions or disorders involving them, you can now recognize various signs and symptoms of injury revealed through a careful, systematic evaluation of these areas. Common principles and basic tests are outlined below that can aid you, as an examiner, to better assess acute trauma and to determine whether or not it is an urgent or non urgent condition.

When thoracic injury occurs, begin your evaluation with the primary survey. To conduct the primary survey, first assess the athlete for indications of serious injury and approach them in a calm and reassuring manner. For a conscious athlete, this enhances relaxation and helps stabilize the respiratory and circulatory systems. Be prepared to clear and maintain the airway free of potential obstructions such as blood, vomitus, and foreign matter. Once a cervical spine injury is ruled out (see Chapter 10) assist the athlete in finding the most comfortable position for breathing. If necessary, be prepared to provide artificial ventilation or cardiopulmonary resuscitation (CPR) and to activate the EMS. A common pneumonic for the primary survey is ABC (Airway, Breathing and Circulation).

Once your primary survey is completed and you determine that the athlete's condition is not life threatening, you then perform a secondary survey. This survey consists of two elements including a thorough history and a complete physical examination. The history is that part of the evaluation in which the examiner questions the athlete to determine the following:

- Mechanism of injury
- Location of injury
- Quantity and quality of pain
- Activities that make the pain better or worse
- Type and location of any abnormal sensations
- Onset of symptoms such as nausea, weakness, dyspnea (shortness of breath), progression of signs and symptoms

The physical examination is your next step. Remember, physical findings may vary tremendously from athlete to athlete, yet still be within their own "normal" range. That's why it's nice to have a preseason baseline exam prior to activity for comparison. Factors such as physical activity, conditioning and acclimatization may account for this variance. Some signs that commonly vary include the following:

- Heart rate (pulse)
- Bradycardia: resting heart rate <60 bpm
- Tachycardia: resting heart rate >100 bpm
- Respiratory rate
- Bradypnea: <12 rpm
- Tachypnea: >20 rpm
- Blood pressure
- Body temperature

It's essential to monitor these **vital signs**. Once you have done so, you then turn your attention to any **symptoms** of injury as your physical exam progresses to the following:

- Inspection (looking)
- Auscultation (listening)
- Percussion (tapping)
- Palpation (feeling)
- Special tests

During the inspection stage of your exam, observe the following:
- Changes in level of consciousness
- Skin color
- Respiratory rate, rhythm, and effort
- Symmetry of chest appearance and movement (flail chest, tracheal deviation)
- Hemoptysis (coughing up blood)
- Vomiting
- Hematemisis (vomiting up blood)
- Ecchymosis (escaping of blood into the tissue or bruising) particularly in gravity dependent portions of the body away from the point of impact such as the flanks, as this may indicate retroperitoneal bleeding
- Athlete's positions, movements, guarding, apprehension
- Cyanosis (pale or bluish skin color of the lips, fingertips, etc.) indicates respiratory distress or poor oxygenation of the blood
- Jugular venous distention (JVD) may indicate tension pneumothorax or pericardial tamponade
- Pupil equality and responsiveness
- Evidence of penetrating trauma

Auscultation

Auscultation is the process of listening for sounds produced in the thorax and abdomen utilizing a stethoscope. Medical professionals with extensive training and experience in this complex skill typically perform this. The specific techniques of auscultation are beyond the scope of this text but they are used to determine the following:
- Presence of normal versus abnormal sounds of the abdomen and chest
- Symmetry or equality of breath sounds
- Respiratory rate and effort
- Depth of breaths

Percussion

Percussion is the process of tapping on certain areas of the body and eliciting certain sounds. These techniques also take extensive training to perfect and are beyond the scope of this text. They are used to determine the following:
- Tympany (indicates air in a body cavity)
- Dullness (indicates presence of a solid organ or mass)
- Hyperresonance (indicates fluid in a body cavity)

Palpation

Palpation is the act of laying your hands on the athlete and determining if there is any particular or substantial injury. It can be used to determine the following:
- General or specific areas of tenderness
- Location of deformities (flail chest, fractures, hernias)
- Location and extent of swelling
- Air crepitus (air trapped in subcutaneous tissue also known as subcutaneous emphysema) often indicates either a pneumothorax or a severe, gas-forming infection

- Bony crepitus (produced by rough edges of bone rubbing together) indicates a fracture
- Asymmetry
- Muscle rigidity (involuntary guarding)
- Voluntary guarding
- Rebound tenderness

Palpation is particularly important in the assessment of the abdomen and it must be used in conjunction with a basic working knowledge of the anatomy, as outlined above, in order to rule out an acute surgical abdomen. When examining the abdomen you must inspect and palpate all four quadrants (again auscultation and percussion are reserved for medical professionals). An acute abdomen can result from the following:

- Internal bleeding
- Leakage of bowel content due to perforation
- Ischemia (lack of blood flow) to bowel or other organs
- Preexisting surgical conditions (appendicitis, etc.)

Symptoms

The symptoms of an acute abdomen result from the irritation of the lining of the abdomen called the peritoneum. These symptoms include the following:

- **Rebound tenderness** is identified by the examiner as he presses slowly and deeply into the abdominal cavity and then quickly releases, allowing the abdominal wall to "rebound" back to its original position. If this procedure is painful, peritoneal irritation may be present.
- **Voluntary guarding** occurs when the athlete purposefully tries to prevent the examiner from pressing on their abdomen due to fear of pain.
- **Rigidity** (involuntary guarding) of the abdominal wall musculature occurs when peritoneal irritation is so advanced that there is reflex spasm of the muscles, producing a board-like hardness, thus preventing the examiner from performing deep palpation.

Other examination techniques used to illicit peritonitis include the following:

- **Iliopsoas test:** Moving leg into hip flexion will cause pain.
- **Obturator test:** With hip and knee in 90-degree flexion, internal and external rotation of the hip will cause pain.
- **Heel pound test:** With hip and knee in full extension, tapping the heel increases abdominal pain.
- **Kehr's sign:** Pain radiates into the left shoulder and arm due to diaphragm and phrenic nerve irritation.
- **The Valsalva Maneuver** can also be used to illicit an increase in pain or to reveal a mass protrusion if significant trauma has compromised the integrity of the abdominal wall itself.

To perform the Valsalva Maneuver, have the athlete take a deep breath, hold that breath, then strain as if having a bowel movement. Any worsening of pain or certainly any mass protrusion through the abdominal wall is considered a positive test.

Other Specific Assessment Tests

Range of Motion assessment is divided into active, passive, and resistive motions and may be approached from three anatomical planes of movement.

- **Sagittal plane** (divides the body from left to right). To evaluate, the athlete stands and slowly flexes his/her trunk forward to the point where the hands touch the floor or toes. He/she then slowly returns to standing and then proceeds with extension backward.

- **Frontal plane** (divides the body from front to back). To evaluate, the athlete stands and slowly flexes his/her trunk laterally to the right, as far as possible. He/she then returns to the upright position and proceeds to slowly flex to the left.
- **Transverse plane** (divides the body top to bottom). To evaluate, the athlete stands and slowly rotates their torso to the right as far as possible. They then return to center and do the same to left. As the athlete moves his/her torso through these planes, visually note any apprehension, limited range, and painful arcs of motion. While observing the range of motion, ask the athlete to state and describe the location, quality and quantity of any abnormal or painful sensations elicited by the movement.

When assessing thoracic injuries, specifically fractures and/or separations may occur in the bones and costal cartilages of the rib cage. If there is a complete separation or fracture, crepitus, grating and popping sensations may be present with active and passive chest movements. In some cases, active and/or passive stress may be applied to the rib cage to elicit and further appreciate these signs and symptoms. Always use caution when examining the thorax as other associated internal injuries may exist. The following tests may be helpful:

Inspiration and expiration test. The inspiration and expiration test assesses pulmonary function and elicit signs and symptoms of thoracic injury. To evaluate, have the athlete breathe in as much air as possible and hold for a few seconds (compression). Then ask the athlete to breathe out slowly and fully in an attempt to exhale all air from his lungs and then hold this position for a few seconds (distraction). During these breathing exercises, observe and question the athlete regarding the location and nature of any symptoms such as inability to fully inspire, pain during breathing or even guarding and apprehension with respirations.

Anterior/posterior chest compression test. The anterior/posterior chest compression test assesses lateral rib cage bony integrity. The athlete may sit or stand if able. The test can also be done while he is supine or in a lateral decubitus position if not. The examiner places the palmar surface of one hand anteriorly on the chest wall at the level of the affected area. Then he/she place the other hand similarly at the corresponding level posteriorly. The examiner then compresses the rib cage by pushing his hands toward each other. This inward pressure from anterior to posterior will cause the rib cage to bow outward laterally. If this elicits pain and bony crepitus laterally then there is a fracture. If no pain or crepitus results then the athlete likely has a contusion or muscle spasm.

Lateral chest compression test. This test assesses anterior or posterior rib cage bony integrity. Again, position the athlete as comfortably as possible. The examiner then compresses the thorax in a similar fashion except laterally at the level of injury, causing the thorax to bow anteriorly and posteriorly. Once again, the presence of pain and crepitus anteriorly or posteriorly is diagnostic of a fracture whereas lack of these symptoms implies contusion or spasm. Similar compression tests may be useful for evaluation of the pelvis as well. The same basic principles apply.

All injured anatomical structures should be properly evaluated. The purpose of a thorough examination is to enable the allied health professional to properly assess the severity of the injury and to make recommendations regarding medical treatment and possible return to participation.

Common Injuries and Problems of the Thorax

Acute traumatic injuries to the thorax may involve the heart, lungs, great vessels and rib cage as well as the trachea and esophagus. Remember that evaluation of such injuries requires a current First Aid, CPR, and AED certification. As an allied health professional, it is essential that you are trained in current basic life support techniques and are able to recognize and stabilize the following until further help can be obtained.

Conditions Involving the Heart

Myocardial infarction. Myocardial infarction (heart attack) is the result of decreased oxygenated blood flow (ischemia) to the muscular tissues of the heart itself. This can be due to traumatic disruption of the myocardial blood flow but is more commonly the result of atherosclerotic disease of the coronary vessels. Common signs and symptoms include the following:

- Persistent chest pain or pressure unrelieved by rest, position change, or medication
- Breathing difficulty; may be noisier, shorter, faster than normal
- Irregular pulse rate; may be faster or slower than normal
- Cyanosis (bluish discoloration indicative of hypoxia)
- Profuse sweating
- Radiation of pain to the left neck, face, shoulder, arm
- Levine's sign (clinched fist over the chest)
- Hypotension or shock

Cardiac arrythmia. Cardiac arrythmia (irregular heartbeat) can be due to either primary heart disease or a direct blow to the anterior chest, in which case it is often fatal. Death can be averted by a well-trained individual with an AED.

Cardiac contusion. Cardiac contusion (bruising) results from a direct blow to the anterior chest wall and can again lead to arrythmias as well as decreased heart function and increased pressures.

Pericardial tamponade. This is a life-threatening emergency where blood or fluid begins to build up around the heart into the pericardial sac and begins to put pressure on the heart, thereby limiting its function. The tamponade can be slowly or very rapidly progressing depending upon the etiology. Findings include a history of chest trauma followed by hypotension, jugular venous distention (JVD), and decreased heart sounds. Once again, a direct blow can cause this, and the athlete must see a surgeon immediately for decompression if he or she is to survive.

Conditions Involving the Lungs

Pneumothorax. Pneumothorax is the result of air leaking from the lung or from the outside via a penetrating chest wound into the pleural space, or the area between the lung and chest wall. It can be spontaneous (without a known cause) or due to either blunt or penetrating trauma.

Tension pneumothorax. Tension pneumothorax results when enough air leaks into the pleural space that the underlying lung collapses and the heart and great vessels begin to shift due to increasing pressure. This will eventually be fatal if not treated.

Hemothorax. Hemothorax results from blood entering this pleural space. It usually results from a broken rib lacerating an intercostal (between the ribs) artery or the lung itself. It can have the same basic effect and must be treated emergently.

Hemopneumothorax is a combination of the above.

Rib fractures. Rib fractures are common and can result in the above noted conditions. They can also lead to or indicate injuries of other underlying structures.

- Fractures of ribs 1-2 are often associated with substantial impact and possible great vessel, neurologic, or mediastinal injury.

- Fractures of ribs 7-12 may be associated with injury to the liver, spleen, or kidneys. Common signs and symptoms of rib fractures include the following:
  - Pain at fracture site aggravated by coughing, breathing, movement, compression
  - Dyspnea (shortness of air)
  - Bony or air crepitation
  - Contusion or ecchymosis

Multiple rib fractures. These can lead to a flail chest where a segment of the bony thorax is completely disrupted and moves paradoxically with respiration.

Rib sprains and strains. These are also very common. Because rib cage expansion and relaxation is essential for the lung's respiratory function, these injuries can be very debilitating as well.

Asthma. Asthma is an inflammatory condition characterized by bronchospasm, resulting in wheezing and shortness of breath (dyspnea). It can be exercise induced and exacerbated by environmental irritants.

Bronchitis. This is inflammation of the larger bronchial tubes and is characterized by a progressive cough.

Hemoptysis (coughing up blood) indicates possible lung injury.

Pneumonia. This is infection of the lungs caused primarily by bacteria, viruses, chemical irritants, vegetable dusts, and allergens. Symptoms may include fever, productive cough and chest pain.

Influenza. Influenza is a viral illness characterized by an acute, rapid onset of fever, muscle ache, headache, and fatigue. It usually lasts one to two weeks.

Pleuritic chest wall pain. This results from inflammation of the pleura or lining of the lung and chest wall. It can occur due to trauma, systemic infection, malignancy, etc.

Hyperventilation. Hyperventilation is an increase in the respiratory rate resulting in a respiratory alkalosis (high pH) due to an acid base imbalance. Usually caused by anxiety or prolonged activity. Symptoms include dyspnea, numbness and tingling in the hands, fingers and around the mouth.

Common Injuries and Problems of the Abdomen

Splenic laceration. The spleen is the most commonly injured organ in adult blunt trauma. Located in the left upper quadrant near the back of the abdomen. Lymphatic organ that functions to filter out old, dysfunctional blood cells. Some immunologic function. Can live without spleen but more susceptible to certain infections.

Liver laceration. The liver is the most commonly injured organ in childhood blunt trauma and second in adults. Located in the right upper quadrant, beneath the costal margin (ribs). Functions to produce plasma proteins, red blood cells, bile. The liver breaks down numerous drugs and body toxins as well as glucose. This vital organ is also involved in fat metabolism as well as mineral and vitamin storage.

Kidney laceration. Paired organs found in both retroperitoneal areas beneath the lower ribs. Filter waste and produce urine. Control blood volume and effect blood pressure. Loss of both kidneys requires transplant or lifelong dialysis.

Hematuria. Hematuria is the passage of blood in urine.

Inability to void. This can be obstructive or functional.

Grey-Turner sign. Ecchymosis in flank suggests retroperitoneal hemorrhage.

Bowel disruption. This is very rare but possible.

Bladder disruption. This is very rare but possible.

Nontraumatic Conditions of Abdomen

Appendicitis. Appendicitis is an inflammation of the appendix. Usually found in young, more commonly males. Characterized by right lower quadrant (RLQ) pain, nausea, vomiting and anorexia.

Indigestion. Indigestion (heartburn) is imperfect digestion associated with pain, nausea, vomiting.

Stitch in the side. This is a muscle spasm or trapped gas leading to a sharp pain in the side which often occurs after physical exertion.

Conditions that Indicate an Athlete Should Be Referred for Physician Evaluation

- Loss of airway, unable to ventilate
- Continued shortness of breath despite no activity and open airway
- Abnormal chest movements. Unilateral or bilateral, suspected rib fracture costochondral separation, paradoxical, or flail segment
- Decreased breath sounds. Suspicious for pneumothorax, etc.
- Tracheal deviation. Suspect tension pneumothorax
- Jugular venous distention (JVD). Indicates increased thoracic pressure, possibly pneumothorax or pericardial tamponade.
- Severe chest, abdomen, flank, or low back pain
- Findings consistent with possible myocardial infarction (heart attack)
- Signs of shock (hypotension, tachycardia, clammy, pale)
- Circulatory or neurologic impairment (dizziness, weakness)
- Signs of an acute abdomen (rebound, guarding, rigidity, referral)
- Hemoptysis (coughing up blood)
- Hematemesis (throwing up blood)
- Vomiting or increasing nausea (beyond a routine illness)
- Blood in urine or stool
- Fever (unexplained by illness)
- Palpable mass or protrusion of the abdominal or chest wall
- Any doubt or concern about the nature and severity of a thoracic and/or abdominal injury. Remember, it's always better to be safe than sorry! Get it checked out by a physician!

Rehabilitation of Injuries

Before sending an athlete back into competition, the following rehabilitation guidelines must be met:
- Full range of motion (ROM)
- Strength, power, and endurance are proportional to the athlete's size and sport
- No pain during running, jumping or cutting

The sports medicine team should design the athlete's comprehensive rehabilitation program. Some suggested rehabilitation exercises are the following:
- Torso range of motion exercises
  - Flexion
  - Extension
  - Lateral flexion
  - Rotation

- Anatomical plane movement
  - Sagittal
  - Frontal
  - Transverse

- Thoracic and abdominal exercises
  - Abdominal crunches
  - Abdominal lifts
  - Abdominal sit-ups/curl-ups
  - Arm extension
  - Arm flexion
  - Bench press
  - Incline press
  - Pelvic tilts
  - Prone extension
  - Prone push-ups

Included in any rehabilitation protocol are the following:
- Range of motion exercises
- Resistance exercises
- Cardiovascular/fitness activities (walking, stair climbing, running, squatting, swimming, etc.)
- Sport-specific activities (jumping, figure of eights, cutting, jumping rope, etc.)

Preventative/Supportive Techniques

Whether to apply adhesive and/or elastic bandages to an uninjured anatomical structure is a decision the certified athletic trainer will have to make. All injured joints should be supported initially. Below is an outline of taping and wrapping techniques:

Wrapping Techniques for Support
- Hip flexor
- Hip adduction

Taping Techniques for the Hip
- Hip pointer

Taping Techniques for the Thorax and Low Back
- Rib
- Low back

Taping Techniques for the Shoulder
- Acromioclavicular joint
- Glenohumeral joint

Protective Devices

The use of protective devices is beneficial, if they are properly selected, used in the appropriate setting, correctly fitted, properly applied, and used within the rules and regulations of the specific sport. Consultation with an equipment specialist and certified athletic trainer is highly encouraged. Listed below are various protective devices that are commercially available to use as an adjunct or replacement to a taping or wrapping procedure:

- Athletic supporter with cup
- Back brace
- Breast support bra
- Low back brace/support
- Rib protector
- Thigh sleeve
- Shoulder pads
- Sport-specific pads
- Sports compression girdle
- Sternum protector

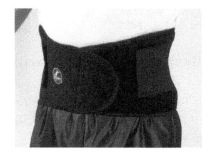

With the interactive supplement, you should be able to view dynamic aspects of joint anatomy (bones, ligaments, muscles), dermatomes and myotomes, PRICES treatment protocol, evaluation format, common injuries, referral guidelines, and knowledge activities (simulation and test questions).

References

American Academy of Orthopaedic Surgeons. (2005). *Athletic training and sports medicine.* Chicago, IL: American Academy of Orthopaedic Surgeons.

American Academy of Orthopedic Surgeons. *Joint motion: Method of measuring and recording.* New York, NY: Churchill Livingstone.

Anderson, M., & Hall, S. (2005). *Foundations of athletic training.* Baltimore, MD: Lippincott, Williams, & Wilkins.

Andrews, J., Clancy, W., & Whiteside, J. (1997). *On-field evaluation and treatment of common athletic injuries.* St. Louis, MO: McGraw-Hill Higher Education.

Barker, S., Wright, K., & Wright, V. (2001). *Sports injuries 3D* (3rd ed.). Gardner, KS: Cramer Products, Inc.

Booher J., & Thibodeau, G. (2000). *Athletic injury assessment.* St. Louis, MO: McGraw-Hill Higher Education.

Gallaspy, J., & May, D. (1996). *Signs and symptoms of athletic injuries.* St. Louism MO: McGraw-Hill Higher Education.

Hoppenfeld, S. (1976). *Physical examination of the spine and extremities.* New York, NY: Appleton-Century Crofts.

Knight, K. (2001). *Assessing clinical proficiencies in athletic training.* Champaign, IL: Human Kinetics.

Lacroix, V. J. (2000). A complete approach to groin pain. *Physician and Sports Medicine, 28*(1), 66.

Magee, D. (2002). *Orthopedic physical assessment.* Philadelphia, PA: W. B. Sanders.

Mellion, M., Walsh, W., & Shelton, G. (1990). *The team physician's handbook.* Philadelphia, PA: Hanley and Belfus, Inc.

National Safety Council. (2007). *First aid taking action.* St. Louis, MO: McGraw Hill Higher Education.

Perron, A. (2003). Chest pain in athletes. *Clinics in Sports Medicine, 22*(1), 2003, pp. 37-50.

Pfeifer, S., & Patrizio, P. (2002). The female athlete: some gynecologic considerations. *Sports Medicine and Arthroscopy Review, 10*(1).

Pfieffer, R., & Mangus, B. (2002). *Concepts of athletic training* (3rd ed.). Boston, MA: Jones and Bartlett.

Prentice, W. (2006). *Arnheim's principles of athletic training.* St. Louis, MO: McGraw-Hill Higher Education.

Rundell, K. (2004). Overuse of asthma medication in athletics? *Medicine and science in sports and exercise, 36*(6), p. 925.

Starkey, C., & Ryan, J. (2002). *Evaluation of orthopedic and athletic injuries.* Philadelphia, PA: F. A. Davis.

Stedman's concise medical dictionary for the health professions (3rd ed.). (1997). Baltimore, MD: Williams & Wilkins.

Street, S., & Rumkle, D. (2000). *Athletic protective equipment: Care, selection, and fitting.* St. Louis, MO: McGraw-Hill Higher Education.

Taber's medical dictionary. (2005). Philadelphia, PA: F. A. Davis.

Thompson, C., & Floyd, R. (2007). *Manual of structural kinesiology* (14th ed.). St. Louis, MO: McGraw-Hill Higher Education.

Weaver, J., Denegar, C. R., & Hertel, J.(2000). Exercise-induced asthma. *Athletic Therapy Today, 5*(3), p. 38.

Review Questions

Short Answer

1. Why is it important to have preseason baseline data (thorax and abdominal areas) while conducting a secondary survey?

2. What are the characteristics of bronchitis?

3. Describe the reason a pneumothorax occurs.

4. If blood enters the pleural space in the lungs as a result of a rib lacerating an intercostal artery, or lung itself, what is the proper name for this condition?

5. Name the four quadrants of the abdominal cavity and a specific organ of concern in each.

6. List the four vital signs.

7. What are the four elements of auscultation assessment?

8. Name the three signs of acute abdominal injury.

9. What is the primary survey for a thoracic injury (pneumonic)?

10. What does the secondary survey consist of?

11. What are the signs and symptoms of a myocardial infarction?

12. Name the two most commonly injured organs in the abdomen.

13. Name five reasons for immediate referral of an injured athlete.

10 Head, Neck, and Spine

Educational Objectives

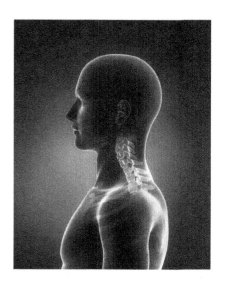

Upon completing this chapter, the reader will be able to do the following:

- Recognize and identify the anatomical structures of the head, neck, and spine
- Recognize the importance of evaluating injuries to the head, neck, and spine
- Describe the steps involved in a proper evaluation of the head, neck, and spine
- Identify musculoskeletal conditions/disorders of the head, neck, and spine
- Recognize common head, neck, and spine injuries
- Explain principles of rehabilitation exercises for the head, neck, and spine
- Differentiate preventive/supportive techniques for the head, neck, and spine
- Identify various protective devices for the head, neck, and spine

Disclaimer on Head, Neck, and Spine

The authors highly encourage all sport professionals to complete the Centers for Disease Control and Prevention (CDC) "Heads Up Concussion" online educational training programs for youth and high school coaches, available at (http://www.cdc.gov/concussion/headsup/). Verification of completion should be available for review by administrators. "When a player shows ANY features of a concussion ... the player should be evaluated by a physician or other qualified healthcare provider onsite using standard emergency management principles and particular attention should be given to excluding a cervical spine injury" (McRory et al., 2013).

Athletic training students are not responsible for stabilizing or transporting severely injured athletes. The athletic training student's responsibilities in emergency situations include the following:

- Recognizing signs and symptoms of serious injury
- Alerting the certified athletic trainer, athletic coach, and team physician of potential dangers
- Implementing a detailed plan to handle emergency transport
- Increasing awareness of the causes of serious injury
- Ensuring equipment and the playing area are safe

Anatomy of the Head, Neck, and Spine

Head

For educational purposes, the head will be addressed in two parts, the cranium and the face.

Cranium

the nonmove-able bones of the head that form the protec-tive helmet for the brain

Cranium. Also known as the skull, the cranium protects the brain from direct trauma but paradoxically can cause injury to the brain during sudden deceleration and can also cause lack of blood flow to a swollen brain after trauma because it is a tight, closed space.

The cranium is composed of distinct anatomical bony segments:
- Frontal
- Parietal (2)
- Temporal (2)
- Occipital
- Sphenoid
- Ethmoid

Face. The face is composed of several, more fragile bones giving us our distinct features. More easily injured but less life threatening:
- Nasal (2)
- Maxillary (2)
- Zygomatic (2)
- Mandible (lower jaw)
- Lacrimal (2)
- Palatine (2)
- Inferior turbinate (2)
- Vomer
- Ear ossicles

Joints. Joints involving the head are:
- Temporomandibular (junction of skull and mandible)
- Atlantooccipital (junction of skull and cervical spine)

The head of an average adult weighs approximately 14 pounds and makes up 9% of the total body surface area. This produces a considerable strain on the cervical spine during physical activity—particularly in contact sports. There is excellent blood supply to the entire head especially the brain and scalp.

Neck

The neck is a relatively fragile area of the body—and, as noted above, it must support a considerable load during athletic activity. Injuries to the neck are not as common as one might think, however, when they do occur they have the potential for serious, life-altering injuries, resulting in either temporary or permanent paralysis or even death.

The neck is composed of the following parts:
- Seven cervical vertebrae (C1-C7)
- Numerous muscles and ligaments (see below)
- Cervical spinal cord with numerous branches
- Major blood vessels including carotid arteries and jugular veins
- Larynx (voice box)
- Trachea (windpipe)

- Cervical esophagus
- Hyoid bone (the ONLY bone in the body with NO ligamentous attachments to any other bone)

Spine

The spine consists of a series of vertebrae that help support the body and protect the spinal cord. The spinal cord contains bundles of nerves derived from the brain that branch out along its course down the body. These nerves control every single aspect of bodily movement (voluntary and involuntary) and sensory ability. It is divided into five distinct regions:

- Cervical (7) as noted above
- Thoracic (12) each attaches to a rib and defines the thorax
- Lumbar (5) attaches the thorax to the pelvis
- Sacral (5) the functional end of the vertebral column
- Coccyx (4 fused) the "Tailbone"

The cervical spine is the most flexible area. It allows for the flexion, extension, rotation, and lateral bending of the neck, thus allowing considerable movement of the head.

Joints. Joints associated with the spine include the following:
- Atlantoaxial joint (junction of C1 and C2)
- Intervertebral joints (junction of all adjacent vertebrae)

The following is a list of terms associated with the head, neck and spine in which you should be familiar and have a working knowledge of the following:

Flexion—anterior movement of the spine
Extension—posterior movement of the spine
Lateral flexion—ear to shoulder
Protraction—anterior movement of shoulders or chin
Retraction—posterior movement of shoulders or chin
Elevation—superior movement of shoulders or head
Depression—inferior movement of the shoulders or head
Rotation—looking left to right around an axis
Sagittal plane—bisects the body into right and left halves
Frontal plane—bisects the body into front and back halves
Transverse plane—bisects the body into upper and lower halves

Muscles of the head, neck, and spine
- Digastricus
- Erector spinae
- Geniohyoideus
- Levator scapulae
- Longus capitis
- Longus coli
- Mylohyoideus
- Obliquus capitis superior
- Obliquus capitis inferior
- Omohyoideus
- Platysma
- Rectus capitis anterior
- Rectus capitis lateralis

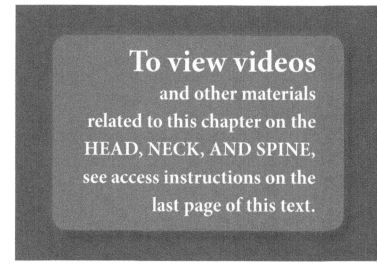

To view videos and other materials related to this chapter on the HEAD, NECK, AND SPINE, see access instructions on the last page of this text.

- Rectus capitis posterior major
- Rectus capitis posterior minor
- Scalenus anterior
- Scalenus medius
- Scalenus posterior
- Semispinalis
- Capitis
- Splenius capitis
- Sternocleidomastoid
- Sternohyoideus
- Sternothyroideous
- Stylohyoideus
- Thyrohyoideus
- Trapezius

Dermatomes: These areas of skin are supplied by a single spinal nerve

C4—upper chest above the clavicle
C5—skin and lateral aspect of arm above deltoid insertion
C6—biceps muscle lateral to the base of the thumb
C7—triceps muscle with distribution to the second and third fingers
C8—intrinsic muscles with distribution to the fourth and fifth fingers
T1—medial aspect of forearm
T2—across upper chest above nipples
T3—across upper chest above nipples
T4—at the nipples
T5—across the upper abdomen
T6—across the upper abdomen
T7—across the sternal notch
T8—across the upper abdomen for abdominal contractions
T9—across the upper abdomen for abdominal contractions
T10—at umbilicus
T11—below umbilicus
T12—groin crease
L1—inguinal region
L2—inguinal region upper two-thirds of anterior thigh (quads) and lateral hamstring
L3—inguinal region upper two-thirds of anterior thigh (quads) and medial hamstring
L4—anteriomedial lower leg and rear one-third of foot
L5—anteriolateral and posterior aspect of lower leg and dorsum of foot
S1—phalanges and plantar aspect of foot
S2—proximal one-third of posterior aspect of lower leg

Myotomes: Level or segment of the spinal cord and corresponding spinal nerve

C2-3—cervical neck rotation
C4—shoulder shrugs
C5—abduction of arms
C6—wrist extension
C7—triceps (extension)
C8—finger flexion
T1—finger abduction

L2—hip flexion
L3—knee extension
L4—dorsiflexion of ankle
L5—extensor hallucis longus (toe extension)
S1—plantar flexion of ankle or hamstring curl, foot eversion, hip extension
S2—dorsiflexion of foot and knee flexion

Evaluation Format

The most important purpose of an evaluation is to determine if a serious injury has occurred. Please refer to Chapter 2 for detailed information on first-aid emergency care, evaluation of life threatening injuries, emergency transportation procedures, and evaluation of non-life-threatening injuries. After a qualified health care professional provider has determined the injury is non-life threatening, an abbreviated injury evaluation format for head, neck, and spine injuries is outlined:

(H) History
Questions should include mechanism of injury, location of pain, sensations experienced, previous injury, loss of consciousness, cognitive function, memory of the injury, and events leading up to the injury (time, place, person, purpose).

(O)Observation
Compare involved to uninvolved anatomical structure, look for bleeding, deformity, swelling, discoloration, scars, pupil irregularity, and other signs of trauma.

(P) Palpation
Use bilateral comparison, assess for potential fractures, note neurological function, circulation, tenderness, deformity, and palpable muscle spasm in the para-spinal muscles.

(S) Special Tests
Assess for neck instability, pain, or weakness in particular area or myotome, lack of sensation in dermatome.

Evaluation of Injuries to the Head, Neck, and Spine

Evaluation of head injuries is of the utmost importance to the team physician, athletic trainer(s) and the coaches. Some head injuries will present signs and symptoms immediately while others may not appear for days. "Any athlete with a suspected concussion should be REMOVED FROM PLAY, medically assessed, monitored for deterioration (i.e., should not be left alone) and should not drive a motor vehicle until cleared to do so by a trained medical professional. No athlete diagnosed with concussion should return to sports participation on the day of injury" (Barton, 2013). All head injuries should be considered major until further evaluation and diagnosis by a physician. Once a diagnosis is reached, the athlete should be monitored for 24 hours and then carefully evaluated on a regular basis for at least one week. The athlete must be cleared by a physician before returning to play or practice.

Concussions
When you hear phrases such as "He got his bell rung," or "Someone cleaned his clock," the individual is referring to the athlete having received a hard hit to the head. These strong collisions or hits sometimes result in a concussion.

According to the Centers for Disease Control and Prevention, a concussion can be defined as " . . . *a type of traumatic brain injury or TBI, caused by a bump, blow, or jolt to the head that can change the way your brain normally works. Concussions can also occur from a blow to the body that causes the head to move rapidly back and forth. Even a "ding," "getting your bell rung," or what seems to be mild bump or blow to the head can be serious* (CDC, 2013).

When concussions occur, the skull is stopped but the brain, which is floating in cerebrospinal fluid, is still moving. This is where the damage (contusion/bruising) to the brain takes place and in turn is when the athlete sustains a concussion. Concussions can occur in any sport that involves contact, either with another player, equipment, or even the ground. When the brain is traumatized, there is a possibility of internal hemorrhaging. An athlete with a concussion is serious because the brain has very little room to swell as it is encased inside the skull. With little or no room to swell and expand, the increasing pressure on the brain will affect the central nervous system, which in turn can and may cause various reactions in the body, including the possibility of the athlete lapsing into a coma or even death.

Concussion

an injury to the brain, usually from the head being hit and the brain shaken

Signs and symptoms of concussions. People with concussions usually fully recover with proper assessment, limited physical activity, and appropriate follow-up medical care. Again, it is important to remember that the signs and symptoms may be acute and appear right away, while others may not be noticeable for longer periods of time. For older adults, young children and teens, recovery may be slower. According to the CDC the following table depicts signs and symptoms of concussions that usually fall into four categories (See Table 10.1).

Table 10.1

Signs and Symptoms of Concussions that Usually Fall into Four Categories

Thinking/ Remembering	Physical	Emotional/ Mood	Sleep
Difficulty thinking clearly	Headache Fuzzy or blurryvision	Irritability	Sleeping more than usual
Feeling slowed down	Nausea or vomiting (early on) Dizziness	Sadness	Sleep less than usual
Difficulty concentrating	Sensitivity to noise or light Balance problems	More emotional	Trouble falling asleep
Difficulty remembering new information	Feeling tired, having no energy	Nervousness or anxiety	

In 2012, a group of experts met in Zurich, Switzerland at the 4th International Conference on Concussion in Sport to develop a consensus statement. In March of 2013, the *British Journal of Sports Medicine* published its findings titled *Consensus Statement on Concussion in Sport: The 4th International Conference on Concussion in Sport* held in Zurich, November 2012, available at http://bjsm.bmj.com/content/47/5/250.full. From their recommendations, a standardized tool for evaluating injured athletes for concussions was updated and titled *Sport Concussion Assessment Tool*, 3rd ed. (SCAT3). A copy of the SCAT 3 for adult (ages 13 and up) and SCAT3 for children ages 5 thru 12 are displayed at the end of this chapter.

Once a physician or other licensed healthcare provider has evaluated the athlete utilizing the standardized tool for evaluating injured athletes for concussions, the decision for further medical evaluation and testing can be decided by the physician. McCrory et al. (2013) reported that there are a number of new technologies that exist to assess concussions (but not limited to) iPhone/smart phone apps, quantitative electroencephalography, robotics-sensory motor telemedicine, eye-tracking technology, functional imaging/advance neuroimaging and head impact sensors (p. 7). McCrory indicated at this point, limited evidence exists for technology's role in this setting ". . . and none have been validated as diagnostic" (McCrory et al., 2013, p. 8).

Athletes with concussions need to be seen immediately by a physician or other licensed healthcare provider. Once confirmed that a concussion has occurred, the physician or other healthcare professional can refer the athlete to a neurologist, neuropsychologist, neurosurgeon, or specialist in rehabilitation (such as a speech pathologist). Getting help soon after the injury by trained medical specialists can impact the speed and outcome of recovery.

Post-Concussion Syndrome (PCS)

Post-concussion syndrome (PCS) is a complex disorder in which a variable combination of post-concussion symptoms—such as headaches and dizziness—last for several weeks or even months after the injury that caused the concussion (Mayo Clinic, 2013). If symptoms continue, the athlete should be evaluated with a computerized tomography scan (CT) or a magnetic resonance imaging (MRI). "An important consideration in return to play (RTP) is that concussed athletes should no only be symptom-free, but also they should not be taking any pharmacological agents/medications' that may mask or modify the symptoms of concussion (McCrory, 2013 p. 4). The athlete's return to competition should not be allowed until all symptoms have subsided. A physician must clear the athlete prior to them returning to athletic activities.

Signs and Symptoms:
- Persistent headaches
- Blurred vision
- Irritability and impulsivity
- Inability to concentrate/attention deficits
- Fatigue and tiredness
- Temper outburst and mood swings
- Learning and memory problems
- Frustration
- Personality changes

Intracranial Hemorrhage

Intracranial hemorrhage is the leading cause of death due to athletic head injuries. There are four types of intracranial hemorrhage, all of which can be fatal. They are epidural, subdural, intracerebral, and subarachnoid. It is imperative that the attending physician, certified athletic trainer(s), or coaches conduct a through evaluation and make an accurate assessment with an immediate referral of all head injuries.

Epidural Hematoma

An epidural hematoma is usually the most rapidly progressing intracranial hemorrhage. It can reach fatal size in as little as 30 minutes to an hour. It is frequently associated with a fracture of the temporal bone and results from a tear of the artery supplying the dura (covering) of the brain. The athlete may have a lucid interval, initially remaining conscious or regaining consciousness after the head trauma before starting to experience progressive deterioration as the clot accumulates and intracranial pressure continues to increase.

Subdural Hematoma

Subdural hematomas are the most common athletic head injuries that result in death. This injury occurs between the surface of the brain and the dura. It often results from a torn venous sinus artery on the surface of the brain. Occasionally, a subdural hematoma may continue to develop over a period of days or weeks and the athlete will often complain that things are "not quite right." When the certified athletic trainer(s), parents of the athlete or coaches hear this type of statement, they need to refer the athlete to a physician for a computerized axial tomography (CAT) scan to determine the continued extent of the injury. With a subdural hematoma that progresses rapidly, and if the athlete loses consciousness, they usually do not regain consciousness.

Intracerebral Hematoma

The intracerebral hematoma is not usually associated with an interval of lucidity and may be rapidly progressive. With this injury, the bleeding is into the brain and is usually from a torn artery and may result from the rupture of a congenital vascular lesion (e.g., aneurysm or arteriovenous malformation). Occasionally, death occurs before the injured athlete can be moved to a hospital.

Subarachnoid Hemorrhage

Subarachnoid hemorrhages are usually confined to the surface of the brain. They are the result of disruption of the tiny surface brain vessels. Like the intracerebral hematoma there is often swelling of the brain, which can result from a ruptured cerebral aneurysm or an arteriovenous malformation. However, because bleeding is superficial, surgery is not usually required.

In review, it is important to remember that all athletic head injuries should be taken seriously and be referred to a physician for evaluation and follow-up care. No athlete should be allowed to return to play without physician approval. For updated information, the authors recommend that you review the CDC website on concussion (http://www.cdc.gov/concussion/sports/ and other professional medical organizations position statement on sport concussions.

Assessment Tests

A physician MUST evaluate all injuries to the head, neck and spine. The purpose of a thorough evaluation is to enable the allied health professional to properly assess the severity of the injury and to make recommendations regarding treatment and possible return to participation. NATA has released a position on the spine injured athlete. This position statement details the appropriate care that should be given to any spine-injured athlete and can be located at www.nata.org. Listed below is an outline of potential evaluation techniques utilized in the evaluation of head, neck, and spine injuries:

Vital Signs
- Pulse: heart rate
- Respiratory rate: breathing rate
- Respiratory effort: effort and pattern of breathing
- Blood pressure: contraction and relaxation of heart
- Pupils: accommodation to sensory input (light, stimuli, etc.)
- Memory: ability to recall facts, situations

Neurological
- Sensory: assess sensory nerves through touch (dermatomes)
- Motor: assess motor nerves through movement (myotomes)

Head Concussion
- Concussion Recognition Scale
- SCAT3 (Sport Concussion Assessment Tool 3, for ages 13 and older)

- Modified Version SCAT3 (for children ages 5 to 12)
- Glasgow Coma Scale: a rating scale to determine the severity of injury
- Romberg: test for proprioception/balance
- Stork stand: test for proprioception/balance
- Heel/toe walking: test for proprioception/balance
- Finger to nose: test for hand/eye coordination
- Memory: ability to recall facts and situations; cognitive tests (state the following: months backward, numbers backwards, remember three words, etc.)
- Eye tracking: ability of eyes to move
- Peripheral vision: ability to view objects in various planes
- Pupillary reflex: accommodate to sensory input (light, stimuli, etc)

Bone Integrity
- Palpation: touching of anatomical structures (physical inspection)
- Distraction: light/mild traction to suspect injured anatomical structures
- Compression: light/mild compression to suspect injured anatomical structures

Special Tests
- Valsalva test: test to increase intrathecal pressure
- Swallowing test: swallow test to determine if pain causes cervical spine discomfort
- Adson test (Halstead): test used to determine the state of the subclavian artery

Common Injuries to the Head, Neck, and Spine

Cervical Fractures and Dislocations

The mechanism of injury is any force that compresses, hyperflexes, hyperextends, or rotates the neck beyond its normal range of motion. These movements can occur in any sport. However they are most common in high contact sports. Symptoms of a cervical fracture or dislocation include the following:
- Pain in the cervical region or back
- Paralysis below the site of the fracture
- Numbness, tingling, or burning sensation in the extremities
- Muscle spasm and swelling
- Decreased limb strength
- Deformity in the cervical area
- History of potential serious injury mechanism

Any history of forced flexion or hyperextension, whiplash, forced rotation, or a hard head-on blow should alert the certified athletic trainer or coach to the possibility of a fracture or dislocation of the cervical vertebrae. Prevention of neck injuries depends a great deal on the athlete using safe and proper techniques. Neck strength and flexibility, as well as proper protective equipment, can also help prevent neck injuries. If a cervical injury is suspected, emergency medical help should be summoned quickly and the athlete should be stabilized. **Never allow removal of a football helmet from a player with a possible neck injury.** Also, remember that the athlete may not have neck pain with a neck injury.

Cervical Nerve Stretch Syndrome (Brachial Plexus)

A cervical injury often seen in football is the stretching or compression of one or more of the brachial plexus nerves. This nerve group begins in the neck and innervates the upper extremities. A common name for this injury is a "burner" or "stinger." When the brachial plexus becomes stretched or contused, a burning sensation is produced that extends from the point of injury into the arm. This condition is typically only seen on one side. A temporary loss of function and some numbness of the arm may also result. The mechanism of injury is usually forced lateral movement of the head or downward force on shoulder. An athlete who has suffered from cervical nerve stretch syndrome must be removed from competition and evaluated by a physician. Even though symptoms may disappear rapidly, an examination is needed to rule out a more serious injury. Medical clearance by the physician must be obtained before further athletic participation is permitted.

Back Injuries

The most common back injuries are strains, sprains and contusions. Sudden, forceful twisting movements, a direct blow, improper mechanics, or a lack of flexibility often causes these injuries. If a serious injury is suspected, highly qualified medical personnel (emergency medical personnel) should transport the athlete for evaluation. Mishandling of a vertebral fracture can cause spinal cord damage possibly resulting in paralysis. Chronic back sprains and strains are common with individuals who have physically active lifestyles. There are very few movements in sports that do not use the muscles of the back in some degree of flexion, extension, lateral flexion, or rotation. When the back muscles are injured, all of the movements just mentioned will produce some degree of discomfort in the athlete. Even the maintenance of normal posture can be uncomfortable. Any injury to the back should be treated conservatively with protection, rest, and medical evaluation. The sports medicine team may use ice, heat, stretching and nonsteroidal anti-inflammatory drugs (NSAIDS) as part of the treatment plan.

Epistaxis (Nosebleed)

A nosebleed is a common injury in athletics, and is usually the result of a direct blow. Concussion is also a consideration when there is a direct blow to the nose area. There are many first-aid methods, which can stop the bleeding quickly. One method is to have the athlete sit up, pinching the affected nostril(s) closed. A cold pack should be held over the nose. The athlete's head should be tilted forward. Tilting the head back will cause the blood to drip into the throat. Bleeding should stop within five minutes. If the bleeding does not stop after using this method, the use of a rolled-up sterile gauze pad or a nose plug can be used to plug the nose. The use of a cold pack should be reapplied.

Eye Contusion

All injuries to the eyes must be taken seriously. If the contusion is severe enough, vision could be affected permanently. A concussion should be considered when there is a sharp blow to the area around the eye. Fortunately, most eye contusions are minor. Capillary bleeding can produce discoloration, or the familiar "black eye." Despite swelling of tissue, the vision remains normal in minor contusions. Signs of more serious contusions include blurred, double or spotty vision, and pain. Blood in the eye is also an indication of serious injury. In such cases, eyes should be patched to reduce movement, a cold pack should be applied, and the athlete should be taken for physician evaluation. Note: Chemical cold packs should never be used around the eyes because of the danger of the pack leaking.

Foreign Body in the Eye

When a foreign object gets into a person's eye, the natural response is to rub the eye. However, rubbing the eye can cause two problems. First, the object may scratch the eye, creating greater discomfort and damage. Second, the object may become embedded in the tissue of the eye, making it more difficult to remove. In removing a foreign body from the surface of the eye: Pull down the lower eyelid and see if that will uncover the object. If found, remove it with a sterile gauze. If the object is under the upper lid, have the athlete look down, grasp the eyelashes of the upper lid and pull the upper lid forward and down over the lower lid. It is possible that this may dislodge the object. If unsuccessful, try flushing the eye with sterile water, applying a protective dressing over both eyes and referring for physician evaluation.

Dental Injuries

Most dental injuries and conditions can be painful and/or distracting, but generally do not require emergency treatment. Simple first-aid measures usually suffice until the athlete can see a dentist. A dentist should be part of the sports medicine program. Reviewing first-aid and emergency treatment procedures with the dentist in the off-season will help the athletic trainer and coach be prepared for common dental problems. A mouthpiece will reduce the incidence of concussion and dental injuries by cushioning the teeth from the shock of blows to the jaw. Mouthpieces are effective in reducing occurrence of dental injuries. They can also help reduce the incident of a broken jawbone—symptoms of which would include pain upon movement, bleeding around the teeth and an abnormal bite. Athletes in other contact sports, such as basketball and field hockey, could also benefit from wearing protective mouth guards. Mouthpieces should be comfortable so athletes will wear them. The coach or athletic training student should inspect them regularly for wear. Worn mouthpieces must be replaced immediately to help prevent dental injuries.

Rehabilitation

Sending an athlete back to competition before healing is complete leaves the player susceptible to re-injury and/or further complicating the rehabilitation process. The best way to determine when healing is complete is by the absence of pain during stressful activity and by the return of full range of motion and strength, power, and endurance to the affected muscle group. Prior to the beginning of any rehabilitation exercise program, the athletic trainer should consult with the sports medicine team to establish an individual program tailored for that individual athlete and the specific injury to be rehabilitated. The following list of exercises can be used as rehabilitative or preventive exercises.

Range of Motion Exercises

Head and Neck
- Flexion and extension
- Rotation
- Lateral flexion
- Protraction and retraction

Spine/Back
- Flexion and extension
- Lateral flexion
- Rotation

Torso
- Sagittal plane movement
- Transverse plane movement
- Frontal plane movement

Strengthening Exercises

Head/Neck
- Shoulder shrugs
- Shoulder/upper arm
- Non-gravity pendulum movements
- Shoulder wheel
- Towel routine
- Swimming

- Light throwing
- Rowing
- Push-ups
- Military press

Spine/Back
- Pelvis tilt (prone and supine)
- Back flexion exercises
- Back extension exercises

Included in any rehabilitation protocol is the following:
- Range of motion exercises
- Resistance exercises
- Cardiovascular/fitness activities (lifting, walking, running, swimming, cycling, etc.)
- Sport-specific activities

Preventive/Supportive Techniques

Taping and wrapping techniques utilized for prevention and support of head, neck, and spine are minimal. Listed below are preventive/supportive techniques for the thorax and low back that provide support to the head, neck, and spine:
- Taping techniques for the thorax
- Ribs
- Low back

Protective Devices

The use of protective devices are beneficial, if they are properly selected, used in the appropriate setting, correctly fitted, properly applied, and used within the rules and guidelines of the specific sport. Consultation with an equipment specialist and certified athletic trainer is highly encouraged. The certified athletic trainer and/or athletic training student would not remove the helmet or neck roll (if used) in any suspected injuries to the head or neck. If a non-breathing situation with the athlete exists, the certified athletic trainer might consider a face mask removal option prior to performing CPR. Listed next are various protective devices that are commercially available to use as an adjunct or replacement to taping or wrapping procedures.

Head
- Earplugs
- Eye shields guards
- Eye shield goggles
- Face shields and masks
- Helmet with face shield
- Intra-oral tooth protector
- Mouth pieces (single, double, lip cover)
- Stock
- Mouth formed
- Custom made
- Nose guards

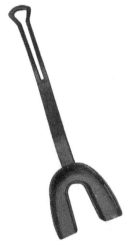

- Nose plugs
- Eyewear, polycarbonate (Lightweight, scratch, and impact resistant)
- Rubber caps for football helmets
- Ski mask
- Sunglasses
- Throat guard that attaches to face protector

Neck
- Cervical collars
- Neck roll
- Neck collar
- Neck straps
- Throat protector

Summary

Injuries to the head, neck, and spine should be taken seriously! When a player shows any signs of a head, neck, or spine injury, there should be a thorough examination by a physician or other licensed healthcare provider. If the player is wearing any type of helmet or headgear, do not remove the helmet or headgear until instructed by a physician, a licensed health care provider, and/or emergency medical services personnel. Prior to return to normal activity, written approval by a physician must be provided and received.

As stated throughout the chapter, no athlete should be allowed to return to play without physician approval. Also, the authors highly encourage all sport professionals to annually complete educational program on sport safety and documents completion of training programs with administrators.

SCAT3™

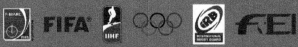

Sport Concussion Assessment Tool – 3rd Edition
For use by medical professionals only

Name _____   Date/Time of Injury: _____   Examiner: _____
Date of Assessment: _____

What is the SCAT3?[1]
The SCAT3 is a standardized tool for evaluating injured athletes for concussion and can be used in athletes aged from 13 years and older. It supersedes the original SCAT and the SCAT2 published in 2005 and 2009, respectively[2]. For younger persons, ages 12 and under, please use the Child SCAT3. The SCAT3 is designed for use by medical professionals. If you are not qualified, please use the Sport Concussion Recognition Tool[1]. Preseason baseline testing with the SCAT3 can be helpful for interpreting post-injury test scores.

Specific instructions for use of the SCAT3 are provided on page 3. If you are not familiar with the SCAT3, please read through these instructions carefully. This tool may be freely copied in its current form for distribution to individuals, teams, groups and organizations. Any revision or any reproduction in a digital form requires approval by the Concussion in Sport Group.
NOTE: The diagnosis of a concussion is a clinical judgment, ideally made by a medical professional. The SCAT3 should not be used solely to make, or exclude, the diagnosis of concussion in the absence of clinical judgement. An athlete may have a concussion even if their SCAT3 is "normal".

What is a concussion?
A concussion is a disturbance in brain function caused by a direct or indirect force to the head. It results in a variety of non-specific signs and/or symptoms (some examples listed below) and most often does not involve loss of consciousness. Concussion should be suspected in the presence of **any one or more** of the following:

- Symptoms (e.g., headache), or
- Physical signs (e.g., unsteadiness), or
- Impaired brain function (e.g. confusion) or
- Abnormal behaviour (e.g., change in personality).

SIDELINE ASSESSMENT
Indications for Emergency Management
NOTE: A hit to the head can sometimes be associated with a more serious brain injury. Any of the following warrants consideration of activating emergency procedures and urgent transportation to the nearest hospital:

- Glasgow Coma score less than 15
- Deteriorating mental status
- Potential spinal injury
- Progressive, worsening symptoms or new neurologic signs

Potential signs of concussion?
If any of the following signs are observed after a direct or indirect blow to the head, the athlete should stop participation, be evaluated by a medical professional and **should not be permitted to return to sport the same day** if a concussion is suspected.

Any loss of consciousness?	Y / N
"If so, how long?"	
Balance or motor incoordination (stumbles, slow/laboured movements, etc.)?	Y / N
Disorientation or confusion (inability to respond appropriately to questions)?	Y / N
Loss of memory:	Y / N
"If so, how long?"	
"Before or after the injury?"	
Blank or vacant look:	Y / N
Visible facial injury in combination with any of the above:	Y / N

1 ## Glasgow coma scale (GCS)

Best eye response (E)
No eye opening	1
Eye opening in response to pain	2
Eye opening to speech	3
Eyes opening spontaneously	4

Best verbal response (V)
No verbal response	1
Incomprehensible sounds	2
Inappropriate words	3
Confused	4
Oriented	5

Best motor response (M)
No motor response	1
Extension to pain	2
Abnormal flexion to pain	3
Flexion/Withdrawal to pain	4
Localizes to pain	5
Obeys commands	6
Glasgow Coma score (E + V + M)	of 15

GCS should be recorded for all athletes in case of subsequent deterioration.

2 ## Maddocks Score[3]
"I am going to ask you a few questions, please listen carefully and give your best effort."
Modified Maddocks questions (1 point for each correct answer)

What venue are we at today?	0	1
Which half is it now?	0	1
Who scored last in this match?	0	1
What team did you play last week/game?	0	1
Did your team win the last game?	0	1
Maddocks score		of 5

Maddocks score is validated for sideline diagnosis of concussion only and is not used for serial testing.

Notes: Mechanism of Injury ("tell me what happened"?):
_____
_____
_____
_____

Any athlete with a suspected concussion should be REMOVED FROM PLAY, medically assessed, monitored for deterioration (i.e., should not be left alone) and should not drive a motor vehicle until cleared to do so by a medical professional. No athlete diagnosed with concussion should be returned to sports participation on the day of Injury.

Figure 10.1. SCAT3 for Adults

BACKGROUND

Name: _____   Date: _____

Examiner: _____

Sport/team/school: _____   Date/time of injury: _____

Age: _____   Gender: ▮ M ▮ F

Years of education completed: _____

Dominant hand: ▮ right ▮ left ▮ neither

How many concussions do you think you have had in the past? _____

When was the most recent concussion? _____

How long was your recovery from the most recent concussion? _____

Have you ever been hospitalized or had medical imaging done for a head injury?   ▮ Y ▮ N

Have you ever been diagnosed with headaches or migraines?   ▮ Y ▮ N

Do you have a learning disability, dyslexia, ADD/ADHD?   ▮ Y ▮ N

Have you ever been diagnosed with depression, anxiety or other psychiatric disorder?   ▮ Y ▮ N

Has anyone in your family ever been diagnosed with any of these problems?   ▮ Y ▮ N

Are you on any medications? If yes, please list: ▮ Y ▮ N

SCAT3 to be done in resting state. Best done 10 or more minutes post excercise.

SYMPTOM EVALUATION

3

How do you feel?

"You should score yourself on the following symptoms, based on how you feel now".

	none	mild		moderate		severe	
Headache	0	1	2	3	4	5	6
"Pressure in head"	0	1	2	3	4	5	6
Neck Pain	0	1	2	3	4	5	6
Nausea or vomiting	0	1	2	3	4	5	6
Dizziness	0	1	2	3	4	5	6
Blurred vision	0	1	2	3	4	5	6
Balance problems	0	1	2	3	4	5	6
Sensitivity to light	0	1	2	3	4	5	6
Sensitivity to noise	0	1	2	3	4	5	6
Feeling slowed down	0	1	2	3	4	5	6
Feeling like "in a fog"	0	1	2	3	4	5	6
"Don't feel right"	0	1	2	3	4	5	6
Difficulty concentrating	0	1	2	3	4	5	6
Difficulty remembering	0	1	2	3	4	5	6
Fatigue or low energy	0	1	2	3	4	5	6
Confusion	0	1	2	3	4	5	6
Drowsiness	0	1	2	3	4	5	6
Trouble falling asleep	0	1	2	3	4	5	6
More emotional	0	1	2	3	4	5	6
Irritability	0	1	2	3	4	5	6
Sadness	0	1	2	3	4	5	6
Nervous or Anxious	0	1	2	3	4	5	6

Total number of symptoms (Maximum possible 22)

Symptom severity score (Maximum possible 132)

Do the symptoms get worse with physical activity?   ▮ Y ▮ N

Do the symptoms get worse with mental activity?   ▮ Y ▮ N

▮ self rated   ▮ self rated and clinician monitored

▮ clinician interview   ▮ self rated with parent input

Overall rating: If you know the athlete well prior to the injury, how different is the athlete acting compared to his/her usual self?

Please circle one response:

no different	very different	unsure	N/A

Scoring on the SCAT3 should not be used as a stand-alone method to diagnose concussion, measure recovery or make decisions about an athlete's readiness to return to competition after concussion. Since signs and symptoms may evolve over time, it is important to consider repeat evaluation in the acute assessment of concussion.

COGNITIVE & PHYSICAL EVALUATION

4

Cognitive assessment
Standardized Assessment of Concussion (SAC)[4]

Orientation (1 point for each correct answer)

What month is it?	0	1
What is the date today?	0	1
What is the day of the week?	0	1
What year is it?	0	1
What time is it right now? (within 1 hour)	0	1
Orientation score		of 5

Immediate memory

List	Trial 1	Trial 2	Trial 3	Alternative word list		
elbow	0 1	0 1	0 1	candle	baby	finger
apple	0 1	0 1	0 1	paper	monkey	penny
carpet	0 1	0 1	0 1	sugar	perfume	blanket
saddle	0 1	0 1	0 1	sandwich	sunset	lemon
bubble	0 1	0 1	0 1	wagon	iron	insect
Total						

Immediate memory score total   of 15

Concentration: Digits Backward

List	Trial 1	Alternative digit list		
4-9-3	0 1	6-2-9	5-2-6	4-1-5
3-8-1-4	0 1	3-2-7-9	1-7-9-5	4-9-6-8
6-2-9-7-1	0 1	1-5-2-8-6	3-8-5-2-7	6-1-8-4-3
7-1-8-4-6-2	0 1	5-3-9-1-4-8	8-3-1-9-6-4	7-2-4-8-5-6
Total of 4				

Concentration: Month in Reverse Order (1 pt. for entire sequence correct)

Dec-Nov-Oct-Sept-Aug-Jul-Jun-May-Apr-Mar-Feb-Jan	0	1
Concentration score		of 5

5

Neck Examination:

Range of motion   Tenderness   Upper and lower limb sensation & strength

Findings: _____

6

Balance examination

Do one or both of the following tests.

Footwear (shoes, barefoot, braces, tape, etc.) _____

Modified Balance Error Scoring System (BESS) testing[5]

Which foot was tested (i.e. which is the **non-dominant** foot)   ▮ Left ▮ Right

Testing surface (hard floor, field, etc.) _____

Condition

Double leg stance:	Errors
Single leg stance (non-dominant foot):	Errors
Tandem stance (non-dominant foot at back):	Errors

And/Or

Tandem gait[6,7]

Time (best of 4 trials): _____ seconds

7

Coordination examination
Upper limb coordination

Which arm was tested: ▮ Left ▮ Right

Coordination score   of 1

8

SAC Delayed Recall[4]

Delayed recall score   of 5

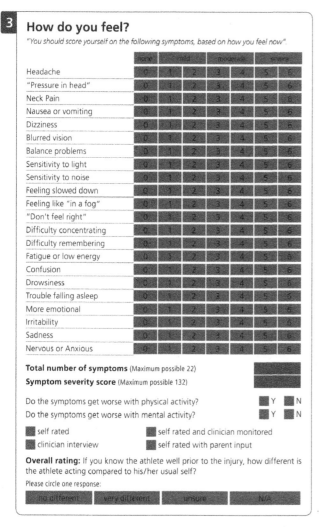

Figure 10.1. cont.

INSTRUCTIONS

Words in *Italics* throughout the SCAT3 are the instructions given to the athlete by the tester.

Symptom Scale

"You should score yourself on the following symptoms, based on how you feel now".

To be completed by the athlete. In situations where the symptom scale is being completed after exercise, it should still be done in a resting state, at least 10 minutes post exercise.
For total number of symptoms, maximum possible is 22.
For Symptom severity score, add all scores in table, maximum possible is $22 \times 6 = 132$.

SAC[4]
Immediate Memory

"I am going to test your memory. I will read you a list of words and when I am done, repeat back as many words as you can remember, in any order."

Trials 2 & 3:

"I am going to repeat the same list again. Repeat back as many words as you can remember in any order, even if you said the word before."

Complete all 3 trials regardless of score on trial 1 & 2. Read the words at a rate of one per second. **Score 1 pt. for each correct response.** Total score equals sum across all 3 trials. Do not inform the athlete that delayed recall will be tested.

Concentration
Digits backward

"I am going to read you a string of numbers and when I am done, you repeat them back to me backwards, in reverse order of how I read them to you. For example, if I say 7-1-9, you would say 9-1-7."

If correct, go to next string length. If incorrect, read trial 2. **One point possible for each string length.** Stop after incorrect on both trials. The digits should be read at the rate of one per second.

Months in reverse order

"Now tell me the months of the year in reverse order. Start with the last month and go backward. So you'll say December, November ... Go ahead"

1 pt. for entire sequence correct

Delayed Recall

The delayed recall should be performed after completion of the Balance and Coordination Examination.

"Do you remember that list of words I read a few times earlier? Tell me as many words from the list as you can remember in any order."

Score 1 pt. for each correct response

Balance Examination

Modified Balance Error Scoring System (BESS) testing[5]

This balance testing is based on a modified version of the Balance Error Scoring System (BESS)[5]. A stopwatch or watch with a second hand is required for this testing.

"I am now going to test your balance. Please take your shoes off, roll up your pant legs above ankle (if applicable), and remove any ankle taping (if applicable). This test will consist of three twenty second tests with different stances."

(a) Double leg stance:

"The first stance is standing with your feet together with your hands on your hips and with your eyes closed. You should try to maintain stability in that position for 20 seconds. I will be counting the number of times you move out of this position. I will start timing when you are set and have closed your eyes."

(b) Single leg stance:

"If you were to kick a ball, which foot would you use? [This will be the dominant foot] Now stand on your non-dominant foot. The dominant leg should be held in approximately 30 degrees of hip flexion and 45 degrees of knee flexion. Again, you should try to maintain stability for 20 seconds with your hands on your hips and your eyes closed. I will be counting the number of times you move out of this position. If you stumble out of this position, open your eyes and return to the start position and continue balancing. I will start timing when you are set and have closed your eyes."

(c) Tandem stance:

"Now stand heel-to-toe with your non-dominant foot in back. Your weight should be evenly distributed across both feet. Again, you should try to maintain stability for 20 seconds with your hands on your hips and your eyes closed. I will be counting the number of times you move out of this position. If you stumble out of this position, open your eyes and return to the start position and continue balancing. I will start timing when you are set and have closed your eyes."

Figure 10.1. cont.

Balance testing – types of errors
1. Hands lifted off iliac crest
2. Opening eyes
3. Step, stumble, or fall
4. Moving hip into > 30 degrees abduction
5. Lifting forefoot or heel
6. Remaining out of test position > 5 sec

Each of the 20-second trials is scored by counting the errors, or deviations from the proper stance, accumulated by the athlete. The examiner will begin counting errors only after the individual has assumed the proper start position. **The modified BESS is calculated by adding one error point for each error during the three 20-second tests. The maximum total number of errors for any single condition is 10.** If a athlete commits multiple errors simultaneously, only one error is recorded but the athlete should quickly return to the testing position, and counting should resume once subject is set. Subjects that are unable to maintain the testing procedure for a minimum of **five seconds** at the start are assigned the highest possible score, ten, for that testing condition.

OPTION: For further assessment, the same 3 stances can be performed on a surface of medium density foam (e.g., approximately $50\,cm \times 40\,cm \times 6\,cm$).

Tandem Gait[6,7]

Participants are instructed to stand with their feet together behind a starting line (the test is best done with footwear removed). Then, they walk in a forward direction as quickly and as accurately as possible along a 38mm wide (sports tape), 3 meter line with an alternate foot heel-to-toe gait ensuring that they approximate their heel and toe on each step. Once they cross the end of the 3m line, they turn 180 degrees and return to the starting point using the same gait. A total of 4 trials are done and the best time is retained. Athletes should complete the test in 14 seconds. Athletes fail the test if they step off the line, have a separation between their heel and toe, or if they touch or grab the examiner or an object. In this case, the time is not recorded and the trial repeated, if appropriate.

Coordination Examination

Upper limb coordination
Finger-to-nose (FTN) task:

"I am going to test your coordination now. Please sit comfortably on the chair with your eyes open and your arm (either right or left) outstretched (shoulder flexed to 90 degrees and elbow and fingers extended), pointing in front of you. When I give a start signal, I would like you to perform five successive finger to nose repetitions using your index finger to touch the tip of the nose, and then return to the starting position, as quickly and as accurately as possible."

Scoring: 5 correct repetitions in < 4 seconds = 1
Note for testers: Athletes fail the test if they do not touch their nose, do not fully extend their elbow or do not perform five repetitions. **Failure should be scored as 0.**

References & Footnotes

1. This tool has been developed by a group of international experts at the 4th International Consensus meeting on Concussion in Sport held in Zurich, Switzerland in November 2012. The full details of the conference outcomes and the authors of the tool are published in The BJSM Injury Prevention and Health Protection, 2013, Volume 47, Issue 5. The outcome paper will also be simultaneously co-published in other leading biomedical journals with the copyright held by the Concussion in Sport Group, to allow unrestricted distribution, providing no alterations are made.

2. McCrory P et al., Consensus Statement on Concussion in Sport – the 3rd International Conference on Concussion in Sport held in Zurich, November 2008. British Journal of Sports Medicine 2009; 43: i76-89.

3. Maddocks, DL; Dicker, GD; Saling, MM. The assessment of orientation following concussion in athletes. Clinical Journal of Sport Medicine. 1995; 5(1): 32–3.

4. McCrea M. Standardized mental status testing of acute concussion. Clinical Journal of Sport Medicine. 2001; 11: 176–181.

5. Guskiewicz KM. Assessment of postural stability following sport-related concussion. Current Sports Medicine Reports. 2003; 2: 24–30.

6. Schneiders, A.G., Sullivan, S.J., Gray, A., Hammond-Tooke, G. & McCrory, P. Normative values for 16-37 year old subjects for three clinical measures of motor performance used in the assessment of sports concussions. Journal of Science and Medicine in Sport. 2010; 13(2): 196–201.

7. Schneiders, A.G., Sullivan, S.J., Kvarnstrom. J.K., Olsson, M., Yden. T. & Marshall, S.W. The effect of footwear and sports-surface on dynamic neurological screening in sport-related concussion. Journal of Science and Medicine in Sport. 2010; 13(4): 382–386

ATHLETE INFORMATION

Any athlete suspected of having a concussion should be removed from play, and then seek medical evaluation.

Signs to watch for

Problems could arise over the first 24–48 hours. The athlete should not be left alone and must go to a hospital at once if they:

- Have a headache that gets worse
- Are very drowsy or can't be awakened
- Can't recognize people or places
- Have repeated vomiting
- Behave unusually or seem confused; are very irritable
- Have seizures (arms and legs jerk uncontrollably)
- Have weak or numb arms or legs
- Are unsteady on their feet; have slurred speech

Remember, it is better to be safe.
Consult your doctor after a suspected concussion.

Return to play

Athletes should not be returned to play the same day of injury.
When returning athletes to play, they should be **medically cleared and then follow a stepwise supervised program,** with stages of progression.

For example:

Rehabilitation stage	Functional exercise at each stage of rehabilitation	Objective of each stage
No activity	Physical and cognitive rest	Recovery
Light aerobic exercise	Walking, swimming or stationary cycling keeping intensity, 70 % maximum predicted heart rate. No resistance training	Increase heart rate
Sport-specific exercise	Skating drills in ice hockey, running drills in soccer. No head impact activities	Add movement
Non-contact training drills	Progression to more complex training drills, eg passing drills in football and ice hockey. May start progressive resistance training	Exercise, coordination, and cognitive load
Full contact practice	Following medical clearance participate in normal training activities	Restore confidence and assess functional skills by coaching staff
Return to play	Normal game play	

There should be at least 24 hours (or longer) for each stage and if symptoms recur the athlete should rest until they resolve once again and then resume the program at the previous asymptomatic stage. Resistance training should only be added in the later stages.

If the athlete is symptomatic for more than 10 days, then consultation by a medical practitioner who is expert in the management of concussion, is recommended.

Medical clearance should be given before return to play.

Scoring Summary:

Test Domain	Score		
	Date: ____	Date: ____	Date: ____
Number of Symptoms of 22			
Symptom Severity Score of 132			
Orientation of 5			
Immediate Memory of 15			
Concentration of 5			
Delayed Recall of 5			
SAC Total			
BESS (total errors)			
Tandem Gait (seconds)			
Coordination of 1			

Notes:

_____

_____

_____

_____

_____

_____

_____

_____

_____

_____

_____

_____

_____

_____

_____

_____

CONCUSSION INJURY ADVICE

(To be given to the **person monitoring** the concussed athlete)

This patient has received an injury to the head. A careful medical examination has been carried out and no sign of any serious complications has been found. Recovery time is variable across individuals and the patient will need monitoring for a further period by a responsible adult. Your treating physician will provide guidance as to this timeframe.

If you notice any change in behaviour, vomiting, dizziness, worsening headache, double vision or excessive drowsiness, please contact your doctor or the nearest hospital emergency department immediately.

Other important points:

- Rest (physically and mentally), including training or playing sports until symptoms resolve and you are medically cleared
- No alcohol
- No prescription or non-prescription drugs without medical supervision. Specifically:
  · No sleeping tablets
  · Do not use aspirin, anti-inflammatory medication or sedating pain killers
- Do not drive until medically cleared
- Do not train or play sport until medically cleared

Clinic phone number

Patient's name _____

Date/time of injury _____

Date/time of medical review _____

Treating physician _____

Contact details or stamp

Figure 10.1. cont.

Child-SCAT3™ F-MARC FIFA IIHF ◯◯◯ IRB FEI

Sport Concussion Assessment Tool for children ages 5 to 12 years
For use by medical professionals only

What is childSCAT3?[1]
The ChildSCAT3 is a standardized tool for evaluating injured children for concussion and can be used in children aged from 5 to 12 years. It supersedes the original SCAT and the SCAT2 published in 2005 and 2009, respectively[2]. For older persons, ages 13 years and over, please use the SCAT3. The ChildSCAT3 is designed for use by medical professionals. If you are not qualified, please use the Sport Concussion Recognition Tool[1].Preseason baseline testing with the ChildSCAT3 can be helpful for interpreting post-injury test scores.

Specific instructions for use of the ChildSCAT3 are provided on page 3. If you are not familiar with the ChildSCAT3, please read through these instructions carefully. This tool may be freely copied in its current form for distribution to individuals, teams, groups and organizations. Any revision and any reproduction in a digital form require approval by the Concussion in Sport Group.
NOTE: The diagnosis of a concussion is a clinical judgment, ideally made by a medical professional. The ChildSCAT3 should not be used solely to make, or exclude, the diagnosis of concussion in the absence of clinical judgement. An athlete may have a concussion even if their ChildSCAT3 is "normal".

What is a concussion?
A concussion is a disturbance in brain function caused by a direct or indirect force to the head. It results in a variety of non-specific signs and/or symptoms (like those listed below) and most often does not involve loss of consciousness. Concussion should be suspected in the presence of any one or more of the following:
- Symptoms (e.g., headache), or
- Physical signs (e.g., unsteadiness), or
- Impaired brain function (e.g. confusion) or
- Abnormal behaviour (e.g., change in personality).

SIDELINE ASSESSMENT
Indications for Emergency Management
NOTE: A hit to the head can sometimes be associated with a more severe brain injury. If the concussed child displays any of the following, then do not proceed with the ChildSCAT3; instead activate emergency procedures and urgent transportation to the nearest hospital:
- Glasgow Coma score less than 15
- Deteriorating mental status
- Potential spinal injury
- Progressive, worsening symptoms or new neurologic signs
- Persistent vomiting
- Evidence of skull fracture
- Post traumatic seizures
- Coagulopathy
- History of Neurosurgery (eg Shunt)
- Multiple injuries

1 Glasgow coma scale (GCS)
Best eye response (E)

No eye opening	1
Eye opening in response to pain	2
Eye opening to speech	3
Eyes opening spontaneously	4

Best verbal response (V)

No verbal response	1
Incomprehensible sounds	2
Inappropriate words	3
Confused	4
Oriented	5

Best motor response (M)

No motor response	1
Extension to pain	2
Abnormal flexion to pain	3
Flexion/Withdrawal to pain	4
Localizes to pain	5
Obeys commands	6
Glasgow Coma score (E + V + M)	of 15

GCS should be recorded for all athletes in case of subsequent deterioration.

Potential signs of concussion?
If any of the following signs are observed after a direct or indirect blow to the head, the child should stop participation, be evaluated by a medical professional and **should not be permitted to return to sport the same day** if a concussion is suspected.

Any loss of consciousness?	Y	N
"If so, how long?"		
Balance or motor incoordination (stumbles, slow/laboured movements, etc.)?	Y	N
Disorientation or confusion (inability to respond appropriately to questions)?	Y	N
Loss of memory:	Y	N
"If so, how long?"		
"Before or after the injury?"		
Blank or vacant look:	Y	N
Visible facial injury in combination with any of the above:	Y	N

2 Sideline Assessment – child-Maddocks Score[3]
"I am going to ask you a few questions, please listen carefully and give your best effort."
Modified Maddocks questions (1 point for each correct answer)

Where are we at now?	0	1
Is it before or after lunch?	0	1
What did you have last lesson/class?	0	1
What is your teacher's name?	0	1
child-Maddocks score		of 4

Child-Maddocks score is for sideline diagnosis of concussion only and is not used for serial testing.

Any child with a suspected concussion should be REMOVED FROM PLAY, medically assessed and monitored for deterioration (i.e., should not be left alone). No child diagnosed with concussion should be returned to sports participation on the day of Injury.

BACKGROUND

Name: _____ Date/Time of Injury: _____
Examiner: _____ Date of Assessment: _____
Sport/team/school: _____
Age: _____ Gender: M F
Current school year/grade: _____
Dominant hand: right left neither
Mechanism of Injury ("tell me what happened"?): _____

For Parent/carer to complete:
How many concussions has the child had in the past? _____
When was the most recent concussion? _____
How long was the recovery from the most recent concussion? _____

Has the child ever been hospitalized or had medical imaging done (CT or MRI) for a head injury?	Y	N
Has the child ever been diagnosed with headaches or migraines?	Y	N
Does the child have a learning disability, dyslexia, ADD/ADHD, seizure disorder?	Y	N
Has the child ever been diagnosed with depression, anxiety or other psychiatric disorder?	Y	N
Has anyone in the family ever been diagnosed with any of these problems?	Y	N
Is the child on any medications? If yes, please list:	Y	N

Figure 10.2. SCAT3 for Children

SYMPTOM EVALUATION

3 **Child report**

Name: _____

	never	rarely	sometimes	often
I have trouble paying attention	0	1	2	3
I get distracted easily	0	1	2	3
I have a hard time concentrating	0	1	2	3
I have problems remembering what people tell me	0	1	2	3
I have problems following directions	0	1	2	3
I daydream too much	0	1	2	3
I get confused	0	1	2	3
I forget things	0	1	2	3
I have problems finishing things	0	1	2	3
I have trouble figuring things out	0	1	2	3
It's hard for me to learn new things	0	1	2	3
I have headaches	0	1	2	3
I feel dizzy	0	1	2	3
I feel like the room is spinning	0	1	2	3
I feel like I'm going to faint	0	1	2	3
Things are blurry when I look at them	0	1	2	3
I see double	0	1	2	3
I feel sick to my stomach	0	1	2	3
I get tired a lot	0	1	2	3
I get tired easily	0	1	2	3

Total number of symptoms (Maximum possible 20)

Symptom severity score (Maximum possible $20 \times 3 = 60$)

■ self rated   ■ clinician interview   ■ self rated and clinician monitored

4 **Parent report**

The child

	never	rarely	sometimes	often
has trouble sustaining attention	0	1	2	3
is easily distracted	0	1	2	3
has difficulty concentrating	0	1	2	3
has problems remembering what he/she is told	0	1	2	3
has difficulty following directions	0	1	2	3
tends to daydream	0	1	2	3
gets confused	0	1	2	3
is forgetful	0	1	2	3
has difficulty completeing tasks	0	1	2	3
has poor problem solving skills	0	1	2	3
has problems learning	0	1	2	3
has headaches	0	1	2	3
feels dizzy	0	1	2	3
has a feeling that the room is spinning	0	1	2	3
feels faint	0	1	2	3
has blurred vision	0	1	2	3
has double vision	0	1	2	3
experiences nausea	0	1	2	3
gets tired a lot	0	1	2	3
gets tired easily	0	1	2	3

Total number of symptoms (Maximum possible 20)

Symptom severity score (Maximum possible $20 \times 3 = 60$)

Do the symptoms get worse with physical activity?   ■ Y   ■ N
Do the symptoms get worse with mental activity?   ■ Y   ■ N

■ parent self rated   ■ clinician interview   ■ parent self rated and clinician monitored

Overall rating for parent/teacher/coach/carer to answer.
How different is the child acting compared to his/her usual self?
Please circle one response:

no different	very different	unsure	N/A

Name of person completing Parent-report: _____

Relationship to child of person completing Parent-report: _____

Scoring on the ChildSCAT3 should not be used as a stand-alone method to diagnose concussion, measure recovery or make decisions about an athlete's readiness to return to competition after concussion.

COGNITIVE & PHYSICAL EVALUATION

5 **Cognitive assessment**
Standardized Assessment of Concussion – Child Version (SAC-C)[4]

Orientation (1 point for each correct answer)

What month is it?	0	1
What is the date today?	0	1
What is the day of the week?	0	1
What year is it?	0	1

Orientation score   of 4

Immediate memory

List	Trial 1		Trial 2		Trial 3		Alternative word list		
elbow	0	1	0	1	0	1	candle	baby	finger
apple	0	1	0	1	0	1	paper	monkey	penny
carpet	0	1	0	1	0	1	sugar	perfume	blanket
saddle	0	1	0	1	0	1	sandwich	sunset	lemon
bubble	0	1	0	1	0	1	wagon	iron	insect
Total									

Immediate memory score total   of 15

Concentration: Digits Backward

List		Trial 1	Alternative digit list		
6-2	0	1	5-2	4-1	4-9
4-9-3	0	1	6-2-9	5-2-6	4-1-5
3-8-1-4	0	1	3-2-7-9	1-7-9-5	4-9-6-8
6-2-9-7-1	0	1	1-5-2-8-6	3-8-5-2-7	6-1-8-4-3
7-1-8-4-6-2	0	1	5-3-9-1-4-8	8-3-1-9-6-4	7-2-4-8-5-6
Total of 5					

Concentration: Days in Reverse Order (1 pt. for entire sequence correct)

Sunday-Saturday-Friday-Thursday-Wednesday-Tuesday-Monday   0   1

Concentration score   of 6

6 **Neck Examination:**

Range of motion   Tenderness   Upper and lower limb sensation & strength

Findings: _____

7 **Balance examination**
Do one or both of the following tests.
Footwear (shoes, barefoot, braces, tape, etc.) _____

Modified Balance Error Scoring System (BESS) testing[5]
Which foot was tested (i.e. which is the **non-dominant** foot)   ■ Left   ■ Right
Testing surface (hard floor, field, etc.) _____

Condition

Double leg stance:	Errors
Tandem stance (non-dominant foot at back):	Errors

Tandem gait[6,7]
Time taken to complete (best of 4 trials): _____ seconds
If child attempted, but unable to complete tandem gait, mark here   ■

8 **Coordination examination**
Upper limb coordination
Which arm was tested: ■ Left   ■ Right
Coordination score   of 1

9 **SAC Delayed Recall[4]**
Delayed recall score   of 5

Since signs and symptoms may evolve over time, it is important to consider repeat evaluation in the acute assessment of concussion.

Figure 10.2. cont.

INSTRUCTIONS

Words in *Italics* throughout the ChildSCAT3 are the instructions given to the child by the tester.

Sideline Assessment – child-Maddocks Score

To be completed on the sideline/in the playground, immediately following concussion. There is no requirement to repeat these questions at follow-up.

Symptom Scale[8]

In situations where the symptom scale is being completed after exercise, it should still be done in a resting state, at least 10 minutes post exercise.

On the day of injury
- the child is to complete the Child Report, according to how he/she feels now.

On all subsequent days
- the child is to complete the Child Report, according to how he/she feels today, **and**
- the parent/carer is to complete the Parent Report according to how the child has been over the previous 24 hours.

Standardized Assessment of Concussion – Child Version (SAC-C)[4]

Orientation
Ask each question on the score sheet. A correct answer for **each question scores 1 point.** If the child does not understand the question, gives an incorrect answer, or no answer, then the score for that question is 0 points.

"I am going to test your memory. I will read you a list of words and when I am done, repeat back as many words as you can remember, in any order."

Trials 2 & 3:
"I am going to repeat the same list again. Repeat back as many words as you can remember in any order, even if you said the word before."

Complete all 3 trials regardless of score on trial 1 & 2. Read the words at a rate of one per second. **Score 1 pt. for each correct response.** Total score equals sum across all 3 trials. Do not inform the child that delayed recall will be tested.

Digits Backward:
"I am going to read you a string of numbers and when I am done, you repeat them back to me backwards, in reverse order of how I read them to you. For example, if I say 7-1, you would say 1-7."

If correct, go to next string length. If incorrect, read trial 2. **One point possible for each string length.** Stop after incorrect on both trials. The digits should be read at the rate of one per second.

Days in Reverse Order:
"Now tell me the days of the week in reverse order. Start with Sunday and go backward. So you'll say Sunday, Saturday ... Go ahead"

1 pt. for entire sequence correct

The delayed recall should be performed after completion of the Balance and Coordination Examination.
"Do you remember that list of words I read a few times earlier? Tell me as many words from the list as you can remember in any order."
Circle each word correctly recalled. **Total score equals number of words recalled.**

Balance examination

These instructions are to be read by the person administering the childSCAT3, and each balance task **should be demonstrated to the child.** The child should then be asked to copy what the examiner demonstrated.

Modified Balance Error Scoring System (BESS) testing[5]

This balance testing is based on a modified version of the Balance Error Scoring System (BESS)[5]. A stopwatch or watch with a second hand is required for this testing.

"I am now going to test your balance. Please take your shoes off, roll up your pant legs above ankle (if applicable), and remove any ankle taping (if applicable) This test will consist of two different parts."

(a) Double leg stance:
The first stance is standing with the feet together with hands on hips and with eyes closed. The child should try to maintain stability in that position for 20 seconds. You should inform the child that you will be counting the number of times the child moves out of this position. You should start timing when the child is set and the eyes are closed.

(b) Tandem stance:
Instruct the child to stand heel-to-toe with the non-dominant foot in the back. Weight should be evenly distributed across both feet. Again, the child should try to maintain stability for 20 seconds with hands on hips and eyes closed. You should inform the child that you will be counting the number of times the child moves out of this position. If the child stumbles out of this position, instruct him/her to open the eyes and return to the start position and continue balancing. You should start timing when the child is set and the eyes are closed.

Balance testing – types of errors - Parts (a) and (b)
1. Hands lifted off iliac crest
2. Opening eyes
3. Step, stumble, or fall
4. Moving hip into > 30 degrees abduction
5. Lifting forefoot or heel
6. Remaining out of test position > 5 sec

Each of the 20-second trials is scored by counting the errors, or deviations from the proper stance, accumulated by the child. The examiner will begin counting errors only after the child has assumed the proper start position. **The modified BESS is calculated by adding one error point for each error during the two 20-second tests. The maximum total number of errors for any single condition is 10.** If a child commits multiple errors simultaneously, only one error is recorded but the child should quickly return to the testing position, and counting should resume once subject is set. Children who are unable to maintain the testing procedure for a minimum of **five seconds** at the start are assigned the highest possible score, ten, for that testing condition.

OPTION: For further assessment, the same 2 stances can be performed on a surface of medium density foam (e.g., approximately 50cm x 40cm x 6cm).

Tandem Gait[6,7]
Use a clock (with a second hand) or stopwatch to measure the time taken to complete this task. Instruction for the examiner – **Demonstrate the following to the child:**

The child is instructed to stand with their feet together behind a starting line (the test is best done with footwear removed). Then, they walk in a forward direction as quickly and as accurately as possible along a 38mm wide (sports tape), 3 meter line with an alternate foot heel-to-toe gait ensuring that they approximate their heel and toe on each step. Once they cross the end of the 3m line, they turn 180 degrees and return to the starting point using the same gait. A total of 4 trials are done and the best time is retained. Children fail the test if they step off the line, have a separation between their heel and toe, or if they touch or grab the examiner or an object. In this case, the time is not recorded and the trial repeated, if appropriate.

Explain to the child that you will time how long it takes them to walk to the end of the line and back.

Coordination examination

Upper limb coordination
Finger-to-nose (FTN) task:

The tester should **demonstrate it to the child**.

"I am going to test your coordination now. Please sit comfortably on the chair with your eyes open and your arm (either right or left) outstretched (shoulder flexed to 90 degrees and elbow and fingers extended). When I give a start signal, I would like you to perform five successive finger to nose repetitions using your index finger to touch the tip of the nose as quickly and as accurately as possible."

Scoring: 5 correct repetitions in < 4 seconds = 1
Note for testers: Children fail the test if they do not touch their nose, do not fully extend their elbow or do not perform five repetitions. **Failure should be scored as 0.**

References & Footnotes

1. This tool has been developed by a group of international experts at the 4th International Consensus meeting on Concussion in Sport held in Zurich, Switzerland in November 2012. The full details of the conference outcomes and the authors of the tool are published in The BJSM Injury Prevention and Health Protection, 2013, Volume 47, Issue 5. The outcome paper will also be simultaneously co-published in other leading biomedical journals with the copyright held by the Concussion in Sport Group, to allow unrestricted distribution, providing no alterations are made.

2. McCrory P et al., Consensus Statement on Concussion in Sport – the 3rd International Conference on Concussion in Sport held in Zurich, November 2008. British Journal of Sports Medicine 2009; 43: i76-89.

3. Maddocks, DL; Dicker, GD; Saling, MM. The assessment of orientation following concussion in athletes. Clinical Journal of Sport Medicine. 1995; 5(1): 32–3.

4. McCrea M. Standardized mental status testing of acute concussion. Clinical Journal of Sport Medicine. 2001; 11: 176–181.

5. Guskiewicz KM. Assessment of postural stability following sport-related concussion. Current Sports Medicine Reports. 2003; 2: 24–30.

6. Schneiders, A.G., Sullivan, S.J., Gray, A., Hammond-Tooke, G. & McCrory, P. Normative values for 16-37 year old subjects for three clinical measures of motor performance used in the assessment of sports concussions. Journal of Science and Medicine in Sport. 2010; 13(2): 196–201.

7. Schneiders, A.G., Sullivan, S.J., Kvarnstrom. J.K., Olsson, M., Yden. T. & Marshall, S.W. The effect of footwear and sports-surface on dynamic neurological screening in sport-related concussion. Journal of Science and Medicine in Sport. 2010; 13(4): 382–386.

8. Ayr, L.K., Yeates, K.O., Taylor, H.G., & Brown, M. Dimensions of post-concussive symptoms in children with mild traumatic brain injuries. Journal of the International Neuropsychological Society. 2009; 15:19–30.

Figure 10.2. cont.

CHILD ATHLETE INFORMATION

Any child suspected of having a concussion should be removed from play, and then seek medical evaluation. The child must NOT return to play or sport on the same day as the suspected concussion.

Signs to watch for

Problems could arise over the first 24–48 hours. The child should not be left alone and must go to a hospital at once if they develop any of the following:

- New Headache, or Headache gets worse
- Persistent or increasing neck pain
- Becomes drowsy or can't be woken up
- Can not recognise people or places
- Has Nausea or Vomiting
- Behaves unusually, seems confused, or is irritable
- Has any seizures (arms and/or legs jerk uncontrollably)
- Has weakness, numbness or tingling (arms, legs or face)
- Is unsteady walking or standing
- Has slurred speech
- Has difficulty understanding speech or directions

Remember, it is better to be safe.
Always consult your doctor after a suspected concussion.

Return to school

Concussion may impact on the child's cognitive ability to learn at school. This must be considered, and medical clearance is required before the child may return to school. **It is reasonable for a child to miss a day or two of school after concussion, but extended absence is uncommon.** In some children, a graduated return to school program will need to be developed for the child. The child will progress through the return to school program provided that there is no worsening of symptoms. If any particular activity worsens symptoms, the child will abstain from that activity until it no longer causes symptom worsening. Use of computers and internet should follow a similar graduated program, provided that it does not worsen symptoms. This program should include communication between the parents, teachers, and health professionals and will vary from child to child. The return to school program should consider:

- Extra time to complete assignments/tests
- Quiet room to complete assignments/tests
- Avoidance of noisy areas such as cafeterias, assembly halls, sporting events, music class, shop class, etc
- Frequent breaks during class, homework, tests
- No more than one exam/day
- Shorter assignments
- Repetition/memory cues
- Use of peer helper/tutor
- Reassurance from teachers that student will be supported through recovery through accommodations, workload reduction, alternate forms of testing
- Later start times, half days, only certain classes

The child is not to return to play or sport until he/she has successfully returned to school/learning, without worsening of symptoms. Medical clearance should be given before return to play.

If there are any doubts, management should be referred to a qualified health practitioner, expert in the management of concussion in children.

Return to sport

There should be no return to play until the child has successfully returned to school/learning, without worsening of symptoms.
Children must not be returned to play the same day of injury.
When returning children to play, they should **medically cleared and then follow a stepwise supervised program,** with stages of progression.

For example:

Rehabilitation stage	Functional exercise at each stage of rehabilitation	Objective of each stage
No activity	Physical and cognitive rest	Recovery
Light aerobic exercise	Walking, swimming or stationary cycling keeping intensity, 70% maximum predicted heart rate. No resistance training	Increase heart rate
Sport-specific exercise	Skating drills in ice hockey, running drills in soccer. No head impact activities	Add movement
Non-contact training drills	Progression to more complex training drills, eg passing drills in football and ice hockey. May start progressive resistance training	Exercise, coordination, and cognitive load
Full contact practice	Following medical clearance participate in normal training activities	Restore confidence and assess functional skills by coaching staff
Return to play	Normal game play	

There should be approximately 24 hours (or longer) for each stage and the child should drop back to the previous asymptomatic level if any post-concussive symptoms recur. Resistance training should only be added in the later stages.
If the child is symptomatic for more than 10 days, then review by a health practitioner, expert in the management of concussion, is recommended.
Medical clearance should be given before return to play.

Notes:

_____

_____

_____

_____

CONCUSSION INJURY ADVICE FOR THE CHILD AND PARENTS / CARERS
(To be given to the **person monitoring** the concussed child)

This child has received an injury to the head. A careful medical examination has been carried out and no sign of any serious complications has been found. It is expected that recovery will be rapid, but the child will need monitoring for the next 24 hours by a responsible adult.

If you notice any change in behavior, vomiting, dizziness, worsening headache, double vision or excessive drowsiness, please call an ambulance to transport the child to hospital immediately.

Other important points:

- Following concussion, the child should rest for at least 24 hours.
- The child should avoid any computer, internet or electronic gaming activity if these activities make symptoms worse.
- The child should not be given any medications, including pain killers, unless prescribed by a medical practitioner.
- The child must not return to school until medically cleared.
- The child must not return to sport or play until medically cleared.

Patient's name _____

Date/time of injury _____

Date/time of medical review _____

Treating physician _____

Contact details or stamp

Clinic phone number _____

Figure 10.2. cont.

References

American Academy of Orthopaedic Surgeons. (2005). *Athletic training and sports medicine.* Chicago, IL: American Academy of Orthopaedic Surgeons.

Anderson, M., & Hall, S. (2005). *Foundations of athletic training.* Baltimore, MD: Lippincott, Williams, & Wilkins.

Andrews, J., Clancy, W., & Whiteside, J. (1997). *On-field evaluation and treatment of common athletic injuries.* St. Louis, MO: McGraw-Hill Higher Education.

Barton, L. (2013). *Sport Concussion Assessment Tool 3.* Retrieved from http://www.momsteam.com/health-safety/sport-concussion-assessment-tool-evaluation-and-management.

Cantu, R. (1994). *Minor head injuries in sports: Proceeding of mild brain injury in sports summit.* Washington, D.C.

Daniels, L., & Worthingham, C. (1986). *Muscle testing: Techniques of manual examination.* Philadelphia, PA: W. B. Saunders.

Del Rossi, G. (2002). Management of cervical-spine injuries. *Athletic Therapy Today, 7*(2), 46-51.

Guskiewicz, K., Bruce, S., Cantu, R., Ferrara, M., Kelly, J., McCrea, M., Putukian, M., & Valovich McLeod, T. (2006). National Athletic Trainers' Association Position Statement: Management of Sport-Related Concussion. *Journal of Athletic Training, 39*(3): 280-297.

Hoppenfeld, S. (1976). *Physical examination of the spine and extremities.* New York, NY: Appleton-Century Crofts.

National Safety Council. (2007). *First aid taking action.* St. Louis, MO: McGraw Hill Higher Education.

Magee, D., (2002). *Orthopedic physical assessment.* Philadelphia, PA: W. B. Sanders.

Mayo Clinic. (April 2013). Post Concussion Syndrome. Retrieved from http://www.mayoclinic.com/health/post-concussion-syndrome/DS01020

McCrory, P., Meeusisse, W., Johnston, K., Dvorak, J., Aubry, M., Molloy, M., & Cantu, R. (2013). Consensus statement on concussion in sport. *British Journal of Sports Medicine, 47,* 250-258.

Mellion, M., Walsh, W., & Shelton, G. (1990). *The team physician's handbook.* Philadelphia, PA: Hanley and Belfus, Inc.

Prentice, W. (2014). *Principles of athletic training* (15th ed.). St. Louis, MO: McGraw-Hill Higher Education.

Prentice, W. (2004). *Rehabilitation techniques in sports medicine and athletic training.* St. Louis, MO: McGraw-Hill.

Starkey, C., & Ryan, J. (2002). *Evaluation of orthopedic and athletic injuries.* Philadelphia, PA: F. A. Davis.

Street, S., & Rumkle, D. (2000). *Athletic protective equipment: Care, selection, and fitting.* St. Louis, MO: McGraw-Hill Higher Education.

Taber's Medical Dictionary (22nd ed.). (2012). Philadelphia, PA: F. A. Davis.

Thompson, C., & Floyd R. (2007). *Manual of structural kinesiology* (14th ed.). St. Louis, MO: McGraw-Hill Higher Education.

Vegso, J., & Torg, J. (1991). *Field evaluation and management of intracranial injuries: Athletic injuries to the head, neck, and face.* St. Louis, MO: Mosby.

Weinberg, J., Rokito, S., & Silber, J. S. (2002). Etiology, treatment, and prevention of athletic stingers. *Clinics in Sports Medicine, 22*(3), pp. 493-500.

Williams, P., & Warwick, R. (1980). *Gray's anatomy* (36th ed.) Philadelphia, PA: W. B. Saunders.

Review Questions

Completion

1. The first seven vertebrae are known as the _____ vertebrae.

2. The brain is protected from direct trauma by the bones of the _____.

3. A _____ is defined as an injury to the brain due to acceleration then deceleration or "shaking" of the brain.

4. A "stinger" or "burner" down the arm is the result of stretching the _____ _____.

Short Answer

1. Name the four types of intracranial hemorrhage.

2. List all components of a comprehensive rehabilitation program?

3. What is the difference in a dermatome and a myotome?

4. According to the CDC signs and symptoms of concussions fall into four categories. Please name them.

5. What was the purpose of the 4th International Conference on Concussion in Sport held in November 2012 in Zurich?

6. Describe the SCAT 3 for adults and SCAT 3 for children.

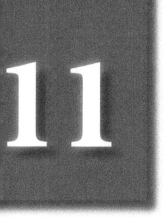

11 Shoulder and Upper Arm

Educational Objectives

Upon completing this chapter, the reader will be able to do the following:

- Identify the anatomy of the shoulder complex and upper arm
- Recognize the principles of rehabilitation for the shoulder and upper arm
- Identify and demonstrate the preventive/supportive techniques and protective devices for the shoulder and upper arm
- Identify the components of an evaluation format
- Recognize the common injuries associated with the shoulder and upper arm
- Review musculoskeletal conditions/disorders for the shoulder and upper arm

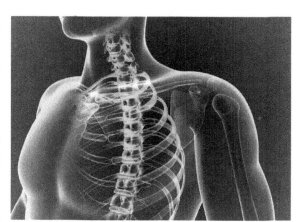

Anatomy

The shoulder is one of the most mobile and vulnerable anatomical structures in the body. The shoulder moves in multiple directions, allowing the upper arm to assume an unlimited number of positions. Naturally, whatever position the shoulder and upper arm assume is yet another position in which they can become injured. The shoulder girdle gains its mobility at the expense of stability. This chapter focuses on two types of athletic injuries to the shoulder and upper arm; those caused by direct and overuse trauma.

The shoulder and arm is made up of these four bones: sternum, clavicle, humerus, and scapula. The articulations of the shoulder include the sternoclavicular (SC), acromioclavicular (AC), coracoclavicular (CC), glenohumeral (GH), and scapulothoracic. The sternum is located on the anterior portion of the body and provides attachment to the clavicle at the SC joint. The SC joint attaches the upper extremity to the torso. The clavicle supports the shoulder complex on the front of the body. There is no muscle or fat covering this bone, so it is easy to feel along its s-shaped length. Laterally on the clavicle, you may be able to feel a projection. On the anterior aspect of the scapula is a bony projection known as the coracoid process. The coracoid process has an indirect articulation with the AC joint through a group of structures known as the coracoclavicular ligaments. Through the coracoclavicular ligaments, the articulation joins the clavicle with the scapula to form the coracoid process, a bony projection on the anterior aspect of the scapula. These two bones are attached in both places by ligaments to form the CC joint. The clavicle does not articulate with the humerus on the lateral aspect but attaches to the medial aspect of the sternum, to form the SC joint.

The humerus is the long bone of the upper arm. The skeletal articulation of the humerus and the scapula is structurally weak, but very mobile. The GH joint is the true shoulder joint and is similar to the hip joint except that the socket is very shallow, allowing for greater movement. The range of motion of the glenohumeral joint is complex and allows for movement in all planes. The scapula "floats" on the back of the rib cage, which is also known as the thorax. This scapulothoracic movement provides critical movement to the shoulder. The scapula, through its muscular attachment to the torso and humerus, has a scapular-humeral movement/rhythm that allows these anatomical structures to move effectively. Another section of the scapula is called the glenoid fossa. This depression articulates with the spherical head of the humerus and is called the glenohumeral joint. The primary ligaments of the shoulder complex allow for the tremendous mobility and movement associated with this region of the body. The strength and integrity of these structures, in conjunction with the muscles, account for the majority of the stability of the complex.

Shoulder girdle

the complex that is made up of the upper arm, clavicle, and the scapula

Like the muscular structure around the knee, the muscles that cross the shoulder's glenohumeral joint add stability to the weak bony structure. These muscles include the deltoid, pectoralis major, biceps, triceps, latissimus dorsi, and the rotator cuff muscle group. The rotator cuff muscle group includes the supraspinatus, infraspinatus, teres minor, and subscapularis, commonly referred to as SITS. The muscles of the shoulder assist with the stability, movement, and strength to this complex anatomical area. The shoulder complex muscles must be strong in order for the athlete to effectively participate in those sports that demand throwing as part of the game.

Rotator cuff

the four muscles that begin the throwing process and then slow down for arm in an overhand pitch

This area of the body is innervated by a number of different nerves. The sensory distribution of a nerve root is called a dermatome, which produces feeling in a certain anatomical area. The motor distribution of a group of muscles innervated by a single nerve root is called a myotome and it produces movement of anatomical structures. Other anatomical structures in the shoulder are known as bursa. The bursae are closed, fluid-filled sacs that serve as cushions against friction over a prominent bone, or where a tendon moves over a bone.

Shoulder and Upper Arm Anatomy

Bones
- Sternum
- Clavicle
- Scapula
- Humerus

Ligaments
- Sternoclavicular
- Acromioclavicular
- Coracoclavicular
- Glenohumeral

Joints
- Sternoclavicular (SC)
- Acromioclavicular (AC)
- Coracoclavicular (CC)
- Glenohumeral (GH)

To view videos and other materials related to this chapter on the SHOULDER AND UPPER ARM, see access instructions on the last page of this text.

Range of Motion: Shoulder Joint

All range of motion definitions are from the anatomical position (standing upright with the arms at the side).

Flexion: movement of the arms upwards toward the front of the body

Extension: movement of the arms backward toward the read of the body

Abduction: movement of the arms away from the body

Adduction: movement of the arms back toward the body

Horizontal abduction: with the arms extended toward the front of the body and parallel to the ground, the arms are moved away from the midline of the body.

Horizontal adduction: with the arms extended outwards away from the sides of the body and parallel to the ground, the arms are moved back toward the midline of the body and toward the front of the body.

Internal rotation: with upper arm at the side of the body or with the upper arm abducted to 90 degrees, the thumb is rotated downward.

External rotation: with upper arm at the side of the body or with the upper arm abducted to 90 degrees, the thumb is rotated upwar.

Circumduction: a full circular movement at the shoulder joint

Elevation: movement of the outer tip of the shoulder upward toward the ears

Depression: the return of the outer top of the shoulder downward toward a normal posture

Protraction: movement of the shoulder blades away from each other

Retraction: movement of the shoulder blades toward each other

Muscles and their Functions

Biceps: flexion and supination of upper arm

Coracobrachialis: adduction; assists in flexion and pronation of the arm

Deltoid: middle fibers (abduction), anterior fibers (flexion, horizontal adduction, internal rotation), and posterior fibers (extension, horizontal adduction, external rotation)

Infraspinatus: external rotation (rotator cuff)

Latissimus dorsi: extends arm; adducts arm posteriorly, internal rotation, downward rotation of scapula

Levator scapulae: elevates scapula, extends and lateral flexion of neck, assists with downward rotation of scapula

Pectoralis major: flexes upper arm; adducts upper arm anteriorly, internal rotation

Pectoralis minor: raises ribs for inspiration, draws scapula forward and downward

Rhomboids: retraction and rotation of the scapula

Serratus anterior: rotates scapula for abduction and flexion of upper arm, protracts scapula

Subscapularis: internal rotation of shoulder (rotator cuff)

Supraspinatus: assists in abducting arm (rotator cuff)

Teres major: assists in extension, adduction, and internal rotation of upper arm

Teres minor: external rotation (rotator cuff)

Trapezius: retraction, upward rotation, elevates scapula, and downward rotation of scapula

Triceps: extends forearm and upper arm

Dermatomes

C4—Upper chest across the clavicle

C5—The skin and the lateral aspect of the arm over the insertion of the deltoid muscle

C6—The bicep muscle lateral to the base of the thumb

C7—The triceps muscle with distribution to the second and third fingers

C8—Intrinsic muscle with distribution to the fourth and fifth fingers

T1—Medial aspect of forearm

T2—Across upper chest above the nipples

T3—Across upper chest above the nipples
T4—At the nipples
T5—Across the abdomen
T6—Across the abdomen
T7—Across the sternal notch
T8—Across the abdomen, supplies motor function for abdominal muscle contraction
T9—Across the abdomen; supplies motor function for abdominal muscle contraction
T10—Umbilicus
T11—Below umbilicus
T12—Just below groin

Myotomes
C4—Shoulder shrugs
C5—Abduction test of the arms (shoulders)
C6—Elbow flexion/wrist extension
C7—Elbow extension/wrist flexion
C8—Finger flexion/thumb extension
T1—Finger abduction

When testing, resistive technique should be used to determine strength of myotome.

Evaluation Format

The first purpose of an evaluation is to determine if a serious injury has occurred. The evaluation format of history, observation, palpation and special tests is thoroughly covered in Chapter 2 and Chapter 6. Listed below is an abbreviated version of this format.

(H) History
Questions should include mechanism of injury, location of pain, sensations experienced, and previous injury.

(O) Observation
Compare the uninjured to the injured upper extremity and look for bleeding, deformity, swelling, discoloration, scars, and other signs of trauma.

(P) Palpation
Using bilateral comparison, palpate neurological, circulatory, and anatomical structures, and assess for potential fractures.

(S) Special Tests
Special tests assess disability to ligament, muscle, tendon, accessory anatomical structures, inflammatory conditions, range of motion, and pain or weakness in affected area.

These tests are well beyond the expertise of an athletic training student.

Assessment Tests

The purpose of a thorough evaluation is to enable the allied health professional to properly assess the severity of the injury and to make recommendations regarding treatment and possible return to participation. Listed below is a review of evaluation techniques utilized by certified athletic trainers.

For further information, the learner should consult chapter references for a comprehensive description of evaluation techniques.

Glenohumeral Joint Stability Tests
Apprehension: detects anterior shoulder instability
Relocation: detects chronic anterior dislocation of the glenohumeral joint
Anterior instability: detects anterior instability of the glenohumeral joint
Anterior/posterior translation: assesses anterior/posterior joint laxity
Posterior glenohumeral instability: assesses humeral head posterior subluxation
Inferior drawer or feagin: assesses humeral head inferior subluxation
Sulcus: assesses inferior instability

Rotator Cuff Impingement Tests
Full flexion (Neers): assesses the presence of biceps tendon and supraspinatus inflammation or impingement
Flexion-internal rotation (Hawkins' Kennedy): assesses the presence of supraspinatus inflammation or impingement

Rotator Cuff Muscular Strength Tests
Supraspinatus strength (empty can test): assesses the strength of the supraspinatus muscle
Drop arm test
Internal rotation strength: assesses the strength of the subscapularis muscle
External rotation strength: assesses the strength of the infraspinatus & teres minor muscles

Internal Derangement Test
Glenoid labrum clunk: assesses the glenoid labrum's integrity and stability

Acromioclavicular Joint Tests
Acromioclavicular joint stability: assesses the integrity of the acromioclavicular and cora- coclavicular ligaments
Piano key or spring test
AC traction test
Cross chest or horizontal adduction: assesses acromioclavicular joint impingement

Sternoclavicular Joint Test
Sternoclavicular joint integrity: assesses the sternoclavicular and costoclavicular ligaments' integrity

Conditions that Indicate an
Athlete Should be Referred for Physician Evaluation

- Suspected fracture, separation, or dislocation
- Gross deformity
- Significant pain
- Increased swelling
- Circulation or neurological impairment
- Joint instability
- Abnormal sensations that do not quickly go away, such as weakness or numbness
- Absent or weak pulse distal to the point of injury
- Any doubt regarding the severity or nature of the injury

Common Injuries

Fractures

Fractures to the clavicle, humerus, scapula, and sternum can occur from a direct blow or indirect trauma (falling on an outstretched arm). In the latter case, the force is transmitted directly to all four shoulder joints, causing a mechanism of injury. The clavicle is commonly fractured in the middle third of the bone, usually resulting from a direct blow. Unlike the clavicle, the lateral end of the humerus is protected by soft tissue. Therefore, with a fracture to the humerus in the shoulder area, the certified athletic trainer may not notice the obvious deformity found with a fractured clavicle. Fractures and dislocations of the head of the humerus should be treated as medical emergencies, because of the danger of tearing or impingement of the blood vessels and nerves that supply the upper arms. When pain, point tenderness, discoloration, and athlete's inability to move the extremity exist, immediate first-aid treatment should include stabilizing the injured joint (applying a sling), treat the athlete for shock, and immediate medical referral for physician evaluation.

Dislocations

The dislocation of the head of the humerus from its shallow socket is common in sports. Injury to a freely movable, glenohumeral joint can occur, in which most injuries result in an anterior glenohumeral dislocation. All first-time dislocations should be considered to be fractures by the certified

Dislocation

an injury to a moveable joint

athletic trainer until X-ray reveals otherwise. A shoulder dislocation is a dangerous condition that should only be handled by emergency medical personnel. A physician is the only person who should reduce a shoulder dislocation. Damage to vessels and nerves can be a problem with this injury. The anterior glenohumeral dislocation occurs when the arm is abducted and externally rotated, a common mechanism during arm tackling in football. Because of the displacement of the head of the humerus, the injured shoulder will look flat compared with the uninjured side. The athlete may hold the arm slightly abducted. With this injury, supporting ligaments and muscles can be torn, causing hemorrhage. Immobilization of the arm in a comfortable position and basic first-aid treatment of protection, rest, ice,

Separation

an injury to a nonmoveable joint

compression, elevation and support (PRICES) should be initiated. Shoulder dislocations require immobilization and a complete rehabilitation program to reduce the chance of re-injury. Since most shoulder dislocations occur with the arm in abduction and external rotation, rehabilitation programs should concentrate on adduction and internal rotation movements. Athletes with chronic shoulder dislocations should be checked by the team physician and rehabilitation exercises should strengthen strained muscles or those too weak for the activities of the sport.

Shoulder Separation

The three less movable joints in the shoulder girdle are the acromioclavicular (AC), sternoclavicular (SC), and coracoclavicular (CC). When injured, these joints are classified as being separated and or sprained and are classified in one of three categories: first degree (mild), second degree (moderate), or third degree (severe).

First degree sprain. One or more of the supporting ligaments and surrounding tissues are stretched. There is minor discomfort, point tenderness, and little or no swelling. There is no abnormal movement in the joint to indicate lack of stability.

Second degree sprain. A portion of one or more ligaments is torn. There is pain, swelling, point tenderness, and loss of function for several minutes or longer. There is slight abnormal movement in the joint. The athlete will favor the injured extremity.

Third degree sprain. One or more ligaments have been completely torn, resulting in joint instability. There is either extreme pain or little pain (if nerve damage has occurred), loss of function, point tenderness, and rapid swelling. An accompanying fracture is possible.

Acromioclavicular (AC) Sprain

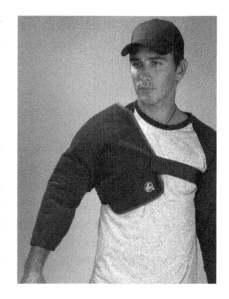

All the ligaments of the shoulder complex can be sprained, but the acromioclavicular sprain is the most common. The frequency of this injury is due to the location of the supporting ligaments. This injury is often referred to as a separated shoulder. The mechanism of injury is often a blow to the top of the shoulder or a fall on an outstretched arm. Depending on the force, the injury can be classified as first, second, or third degree. The first degree sprain mildly stretches the acromioclavicular ligaments, resulting in pain between the clavicle and acromion process of the scapula. There is no deformity. The second degree sprain has some tearing of the ligaments, resulting in clavicle displacement. The athlete will express pain, discomfort, and inability to perform range of motion exercises. Third degree sprains result in extreme pain and obvious displacement of the clavicle. Surgery may be required.

A simple functional test that can be done to confirm an AC sprain is to have the athlete touch the opposite shoulder with the hand of the injured side. If there is an AC sprain, this movement may be painful, and perhaps even impossible to perform, depending on the severity of the injury. Basic first-aid treatment for AC sprains includes protection, rest, ice, compression, elevation, and support (arm sling) along with referral to a physician for evaluation. During the healing process, the sports medicine team can implement a comprehensive rehabilitation program that begins by establishing pain free range of motion in combination with light exercises in order to maintain and increase strength and function. Prior to return to physical activity, selection of preventive/supportive techniques and protective devices can be utilized to reduce the occurrence of re-injury.

Muscular Strains

Since the shoulder has many movements, muscular strains to the shoulder girdle are common. Common causes of shoulder muscle strains are lack of strength, repetitive overuse, improper technique, and inadequate warm-up. When palpating the area, the athletic training students may note soreness or pain primarily in the soft tissue. As the athletic training student resists the athlete's flexion, extension, and other movements, one particular range of motion may produce the most pain. The basic treatment should consist of protection, rest, ice, compression, elevation, and support.

Contusions of the Shoulder

Both the muscles and the bones of the shoulder are often bruised in sports. The lateral aspect of the clavicle is especially susceptible to contusion, commonly known as a shoulder pointer. Once an AC sprain has been ruled out, treatment of the contusion should include the basic treatment of PRICES along with protective padding utilized prior to return to physical activity.

Brachial Plexus

As previously reviewed in Chapter 10, a cervical or shoulder injury often seen in football is the stretching or contusion of one or more of the brachial plexus nerves. This nerve group begins in the neck and innervates the upper extremities. When the brachial plexus becomes stretched or contused, a burning sensation is produced that extends from the point of injury into the arm, often resulting in temporary loss of function and numbness of the arm.

Brachial plexus

the complex of nerves that innervate the shoulder and the arm

An athlete who has suffered from brachial plexus must be removed from competition and checked by a physician. Medical clearance by the physician must be obtained before further athletic participation is permitted.

Throwing Injuries to the Shoulder

Overhead throwing injuries to the shoulder are very common in variety of sports. (baseball, softball, volleyball, javelin, tennis, etc.) Overhead throwing is a high speed, highly ballistic activity that requires careful management and well thought out preparation. Some of the pathologies that can occur due to overhead throwing include: rotator cuff strain or rupture, internal impingement, external impingement, tendinopathy, SLAP (superior labral tear from anterior to posterior) injury, and scapular dyskinesis. Many of these pathologies are classified as overuse injuries and once present must be treated with rest and rehabilitation.

Prevention is a key component for many of these overhead throwing injury pathologies. Some important factors in prevention of overhead throwing injures include the following:
- Warm up to throw (don't use throwing as a warm-up exercise)
- Implement sport-specific strengthening exercises for rotator cuff and scapular stabilization
- Implement a progressive throwing program (progression over time of velocity, distance, and number of throws)
- Get in throwing shape before throwing competitively
- Restrict high pitch counts
- Allow proper rest/recovery (avoid throwing on short rest)
- Don't throw with pain

Musculoskeletal Conditions/Disorders

Listed are musculoskeletal conditions/disorders that affect the shoulder and upper arm. Define and review these conditions using a medical dictionary.
- Blocker's exostosis
- Bursitis
- Contusions
- Nerve injury
- Rotator cuff strain
- Subluxation
- Synovitis
- Tendinitis/tenosynovitis
- Winged scapula

Rehabilitation

Before sending an athlete back to competition, the following rehabilitation guidelines must be met:
- Full range of motion
- Strength, power, and endurance are proportional to the athlete's size and sport
- No pain during functional upper extremity activities (throwing, catching)

The sports medicine team should design the athlete's comprehensive rehabilitation program. A list of suggested rehabilitation exercises are outlined in the next section.

Range of Motion Exercises
- Flexion and extension
- Abduction and adduction
- Horizontal abduction and adduction
- Internal and external rotation—with arm at the side of the body
- Internal and external rotation—with the arm abducted to 90 degrees
- Circumduction
- Elevation and depression
- Protraction and retraction

Shoulder and Arm-Strengthening Exercises
- Non-gravity pendulum movements
- Shoulder fly (abduction to 90 degrees) with dumbbells
- Push-ups
- Rowing
- Thrower's Ten exercise program (Found at: http://www.athleticmed.com/pdf/Throwers_Ten_Exercise_Program.pdf), elastic band exercises for rotator cuff and scapular stabilizers
- Towel movement routine

Included in any rehabilitation protocol would be the following:
- Range of motion exercises
- Resistance exercises
- Cardiovascular/fitness activities (lifting, walking, running, swimming, etc)
- Sport-specific activities (progressive throwing, jumping rope, wall push-ups, lifting weights, etc.)

Protective Devices

Listed are various protective devices that are commercially available to use as an adjunct or replacement to taping or wrapping procedures. Prior to use, consultation with an equipment specialist and certified athletic trainer is highly encouraged.
- AC joint pad
- Blockers exostosis pad
- Deltoid pad
- Glenohumeral joint stabilizer brace
- Shoulder pads (football, hockey, etc.)

Preventive/Supportive Techniques

An outline of basic taping and wrapping techniques is listed. For detailed information, consult this chapter's reference.

Wrapping Techniques for Support
Glenohumeral joint wrap

Taping Techniques for the Shoulder
Acromioclavicular joint

Glenohumeral Joint Wrap

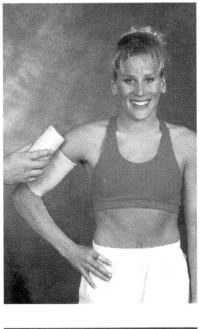
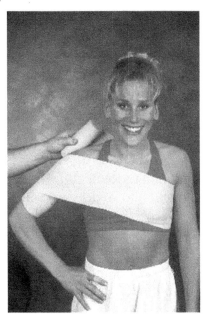
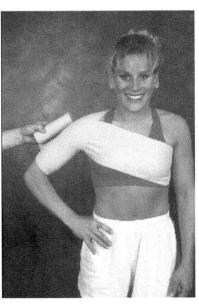
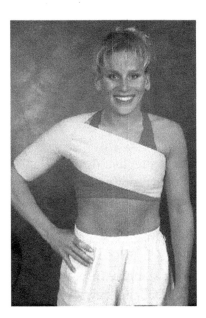

Wrapping Procedures:
1. A continuous strip of 6" elastic wrap is applied in a shoulder spica method. This supportive technique should restrict abduction and external rotation of the glenohumeral joint. Begin on the distal aspect of the biceps muscle of the affected arm, move anteriorly, and encircle the arm.
2. Continue the wrap across the anterior aspect of the chest, under the opposite arm, across the posterior aspect of the torso, and encircle the distal aspect of the upper arm.
3. Repeat this procedure a second time.
4. Secure the wrap by using a continuous strip of elastic tape in the same pattern as the wrap. Anchor the wrap with 2" elastic tape following the same pattern as the wrap.

References

Anderson, M., & Hall, S. (2012). *Foundations of athletic training* (5th ed.). Baltimore, MD: Lippincott Williams & Wilkins.

Andrews, J., Clancy, W., & Whiteside, J. (1997). *On-field evaluation and treatment of common athletic injuries.* St. Louis, MO: McGraw-Hill Higher Education.

Axe, M. (2000). Acromioclavicular joint injuries in the athlete. *Sports Medicine and Arthroscopy Review, 8*(2), pp. 182-191.

Barker, S., Wright, K., & Wright, V. (2007). *Sports injuries 3D* (3rd ed.). Gardner, KS: Cramer Products, Inc.

Booher, J., & Thibodeau, G. (2000). *Athletic injury assessment* (4th ed.). St. Louis, MO: McGraw-Hill Higher Education.

Gallaspy, J., & May, D. (1996). *Signs and symptoms of athletic injuries.* St. Louis, MO: McGraw-Hill Higher Education.

Hoppenfeld, S. (1976). *Physical examination of the spine and extremities.* New York, NY: Appleton-Century Crofts.

Knight, K. (2010). *Developing clinical proficiencies in athletic training* (4th ed.). Champaign, IL: Human Kinetics.

Magee, D. (2008). *Orthopedic physical assessment* (5th ed.). Philadelphia, PA: W. B. Sanders.

Mellion, M., Walsh, W., & Shelton, G. (1990). *The team physician's handbook.* Philadelphia, PA: Hanley and Belfus, Inc.

National Safety Council. (2007). *First aid taking action.* St. Louis, MO: McGraw-Hill Higher Education.

Prentice, W. (2014). *Arnheim's principles of athletic training* (15th ed.). St. Louis, MO: McGraw-Hill Higher Education.

Prentice, W. (2011). *Rehabilitation techniques in sports medicine and athletic training* (5th ed.). St. Louis, MO: McGraw-Hill.

Prentice, W. (2009). Therapeutic modalities in sports medicine (6th ed.). St. Louis, MO: McGraw-Hill Higher Education.

Starkey, C. (2013). *Athletic training and sports medicine: An integrated approach* (5th ed.). Burlington, MA: Jones and Bartlett Learning.

Starkey, C., & Ryan, J. (2010). *Evaluation of orthopedic and athletic injuries* (3th ed.). Philadelphia: F. A. Davis.

Starkey, C. (2013). *Therapeutic modalities* (4th ed.). Philadelphia, PA: F. A. Davis.

Stedman's medical dictionary for the health professions and nursing (7th ed.). (2011). Lippincott Williams & Wilkins.

Street, S., & Rumkle, D. (2000). *Athletic protective equipment: Care, selection, and fitting.* St. Louis, MO: McGraw-Hill Higher Education.

Taber's medical dictionary (22nd ed.). (2013). Philadelphia, PA: F. A. Davis.

Thompson, C., & Floyd, R. (2012). *Manual of structural kinesiology* (18th ed.). St. Louis, MO: McGraw-Hill Higher Education.

Wright, K., Whitehill, W., & Lewis, M. (2005). *Preventive techniques: Taping/wrapping techniques and protective devices.* Gardner, KS: Cramer Products.

Suggested Multimedia Resources

Wright K., & Whitehill, W. (1996). *Sports medicine taping series: The shoulder and elbow.* St. Louis, MO: McGraw-Hill Higher Education.

Wright, K., Harrelson, G., Floyd, R., & Fincher L. (1994). *Sports medicine evaluation series: The shoulder.* St. Louis, MO: Mosby Year Book, Inc.

Wright, K., Harrelson, G., Floyd, R., & Fincher, L. (1994). *Sports medicine evaluation series: The elbow.* St. Louis, MO: Mosby Year Book, Inc.

Review Questions

Completion

1. The_____is the point where the clavicle articulates with the scapula.

2. The clavicle does not articulate with the_____.

3. The_____glenohumeral dislocation occurs when the arm is_____and_____rotated.

4. The four bones that make up the shoulder/upper arm complex are the _____,_____,_____, and_____.

5. The_____end of the clavicle articulates with the sternum. The _____end articulates with the acromion process.

6. _____attach the scapula to the clavicle.

7. Resistance to shoulder movements can often reveal an injury to a specific_____.

8. With a shoulder dislocation, you should always suspect a_____.

9. Contusions to the distal end of the clavicle are called_____.

10. The four deep muscles that stabilize the head of the humerus into the glenoid fossa are referred to as the rotator cuff. The four muscles are:_____, _____,_____, and_____.

Short Answer

1. Name three components of a rehabilitation protocol:

2. Name four shoulder rehabilitative exercises:

3. Name an internal derangement test.

4. Describe the basic first aid treatment for a fractured clavicle.

5. What is a common mechanism of an acromioclavicular (AC) sprain?

6. What is the difference between a separation and a dislocation to a joint?

12 Elbow, Forearm, Wrist, and Hand

Educational Objectives

Upon completing this chapter, the reader will be able to do the following:

- Identify the anatomy of the elbow, forearm, wrist, and hand
- Recognize the principles of rehabilitation exercises for the elbow, forearm, wrist, and hand
- Identify and demonstrate the preventive/supportive techniques and protective devices for the elbow, forearm, wrist, and hand
- Identify the components of an evaluation format
- Recognize the common injuries associated with the elbow, forearm, wrist, and hand
- Review musculoskeletal conditions/disorders for the elbow, forearm, wrist, and hand

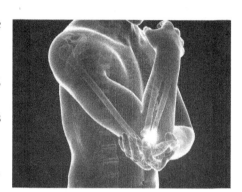

Anatomy

The elbow joint is an intricate collection of bones, muscles, ligaments, and nerves. It permits the movements of flexion, extension, pronation, and supination. Many sports place specific demands on the elbow and each movement can lead to a specific injury. The elbow joint often delivers, and sometimes receives, accidental blows that can cause bruising, fracture, dislocation, or nerve damage. Excessive stresses are placed on the elbow in throwing and racquet sports.

The humerus, the largest bone of the upper extremity, has two articulating condyles at its distal end. Of the two bones of the forearm, the ulna remains stationary and radius rotates on the ulna as the forearm, wrist, and hand pronate and supinate. The proximal end of the ulna has a bony protuberance called the olecranon process. It is the olecranon process that articulates with the proximal radius. While in anatomical position, hanging your arm at your side with the palm facing forward, the small bony prominence at the tip of the elbow. The lateral epicondyle is on the opposite side. When the elbow is bent, the condyle process is observed and easily palpable, as it is the pointed bony prominence bony prominence at the tip of the elbow. Ligaments and tendons use the condyles of the humerus as a base of attachment. The joints of elbow are, the humeroulnar joint, the humeroradial joint, and the radioulnar joint. Within these joints, the ligaments that support this joint are the ulnar collateral, radial collateral, and annular ligaments.

The medial condyle articulates with the ulna of the forearm to allow flexion and extension of the elbow. The lateral condyle of the humerus articulates with the radius. The articulation of the radius and the ulna make up the radioulnar joint and allows pronation and supination of the lower arm and hand. The elbow joint is considered to have very strong ligamentous and muscular support. Medial and lateral collateral ligaments support this joint. The medial collateral ligament is attached to the humerus and the ulna. The lateral collateral ligament is attached to the humerus and the radius. Adding further to the elbow's stability is the annular ligament. This ligament attaches to the ulna and completely encircles the head of the radius. The annular ligament helps keep the radius and ulna from separating.

The muscles that control the elbow's movement originate above the elbow, on the humerus and the scapula (shoulder blade). These muscles include the biceps, triceps, and brachialis. The numerous muscles that control the movements of the forearm, wrist, and fingers originate on the two epicondyles of the humerus. Muscles that allow the forearm to flex and pronate are the flexor carpi radialis, flexor carpi ulnaris, flexor digitorum sublimis, and flexor pollicis longus. Forearm muscles that permit extension and supination are the extensor digitorum communis, extensor carpi radialis longus and brevis, extensor carpi ulnaris, and extensor pollicis longus.

The wrist and hand are the site of some of the most minor, yet irritating, conditions suffered by athletes. Examples of these conditions include blisters, calluses, and acute sprains and strains. These conditions can be disabling if excessive stress is applied. The wrist and hand contain 27 bones (8 carpal bones, 5 metacarpals, and 14 phalanges) and 38 joints. The carpal bones are the scaphoid, lunate, triquetral, pisiform, trapezium, trapezoid, capitate, and hamate. Of the carpal bones, the scaphiod is most commonly fractured, and the lunate is most often dislocated.

The hand region is made up of the five metacarpal bones, and the fingers have 14 bones known as the phalanges. Within the wrist, hand, and fingers, there are numerous joints that allow movement. These are the radiocarpal, carpal, carpometacarpal, intercarpal, metacarpophalangeal (MCP), and interphalangeal, which include distal interphalangeal (DIP) and proximal interphalangeal (PIP) joints in the fingers. The muscles within the wrist and hand include abductor pollicis brevis, flexor pollicis brevis, opponens pollicis, adductor pollicis, abductor digiti minimi, flexor digiti minimi brevis, opponens digiti minimi, palmar interossei, and dorsal interossei.

This area of the body is innervated by a number of different nerves. The sensory distribution of a nerve root is called a dermatome, which produces feeling in a certain anatomical area. The motor distribution of a group of muscles innervated by a single nerve root is called a myotome and it produces movement of anatomical structures.

Elbow, Forearm, Wrist, and Hand Anatomy

Bones
- Humerus
- Radius
- Ulna
- Scaphoid (navicular)
- Lunate
- Triquetral
- Pisiform
- Trapezium
- Trapezoid
- Capitate
- Hamate
- Metacarpals (5)
- Phalanges (14)

Ligaments/Structures
- Elbow
- Medial collateral (ulna) ligament
- Lateral collateral (radial) ligament
- Annular ligament
- Interosseous membrane

Wrist
- Ulnar collateral ligament
- Radial collateral ligament
- Palmar (volar) radiocarpal

Ligament
- Hand and fingers
- Transverse carpal ligament

- Collateral ligaments of the phalanges
- PIP collateral ligaments
- DIP collateral ligaments

Joints
Elbow
- Humeroulnar
- Humeroradial
- Radioulnar

Wrist
- Radiocarpal
- Midcarpal
- Intercarpal
- Radioulnar
- Carpometacarpal

Hand
- Metacarpophalangeal (MCP)
- Interphalangeal: proximal (PIP) and distal (DIP)

Muscles and their Functions
- **Biceps:** Flexion and supination of arm
- **Triceps**: Extends forearm and upper arm
- **Coracobrachialis:** adduction; assists in flexion and pronation of the arm
- **Brachialis:** Flexion at elbow
- **Anconeus:** Extension at elbow
- **Brachioradialis:** Flexion at elbow with thumb up position
- **Supinator:** Supination
- **Pronator teres:** Pronation
- **Pronator quadratus:** Pronation

Forearm Pronators and Wrist Flexors
- Flexor carpi radialis
- Flexor carpi ulnaris
- Flexor pollicis longus
- Flexor digitorum profundus
- Flexor digitorum superficialis palmaris longus

Forearm Supinators and Wrist Extensors
- Extensor digitorum communis extensor carpi radialis brevis
- Extensor carpi radialis longus
- Extensor carpi ulnaris
- Extensor pollicis longus

Wrist/Hand/Fingers Extrinsics
- Flexor digitorum profundus: flexion of DIP joint
- Flexor digitorum superficialis: flexion of PIP joint
- Abductor pollicis longus: adduction of MCP and flexion of MCP of thumb
- Extensor pollicis brevis: abduction of thumb
- Extensor pollicis longus: extension of thumb
- Extensor digitorum communi: extension of MCP joint
- Extensor indicis propius: extension of the MCP joint of the index finger extensor digitorum
- Quinti propius (digitus minimi): extension of MCP joint of the fifth finger
- Flexor pollicis longus: flexion of MCP joint of thumb

Wrist/Hand/Fingers Intrinsics
- Lumbricals I, II, III, and IV: flexion of MCP joints; extension of IP joints.
- Palmar interossei: abduction of digit 1, 2, 3, and 4; flexion of MCP and extension of IP joints of digits
- Dorsal interossei: abduction, flexion, and extension of the above
- Adductor pollicis: adducts the thumb
- Opponens pollicis: opposition of thumb
- Abductor digiti minimi: abduction of the little finger
- Flexor digiti minimi brevis: flexion of MCP joint of little finger
- Opponens digiti minimi: Opposition of little finger

Range of Motion
Elbow
- **Flexion:** decreasing the angle between the humerus and the forearm
- **Extension:** increasing the angle between the humerus and the forearm
- **Supination:** movement of the palm upward
- **Pronation:** movement of the palm downward

Wrist
- **Flexion:** decreasing the angle between the forearm and the hand
- **Extension:** increasing the angle between the forearm and hand

- **Radial deviation:** movement of the wrist to the thumb side
- **Ulnar deviation:** movement of the wrist to the little finger side
- **Supination:** turning the palm up
- **Pronation:** turning the palm down

Fingers
- **Flexion:** decreasing the angle between the joints
- **Extension:** increasing the angle between the joints
- **Abduction:** movement away from median plane, as in separating fingers
- **Adduction:** movement toward median plane of body, as in bring fingers
- **Opposition:** movement of the thumb to touch all other fingers
- **Thumb flexion, abduction and adduction:** carpometacarpal and metacarpophalangeal joints
- **Opposition:** movement of the thumb to touch all other fingers

Dermatomes
C5—The skin and the lateral aspect of the arm over the insertion of the deltoid muscle
C6—The biceps muscle lateral to the base of the thumb
C7—The triceps muscle with distribution to the second and third fingers
C8—Intrinsic muscle with distribution to the fourth and fifth fingers
T1—Medial aspect of forearm
T2—Across upper chest above the nipples

Myotomes
C4—Shoulder shrugs
C5—Abduction test of the arms C6, wrist extension
C7—Triceps (extension) C8, finger flexion
T1—Finger abduction

When determining strength of myotomes, provide resistive force.

- **Nerve sensory:** upper extremities
- **Radial nerve:** web space between the thumb and index finger
- **Median nerve:** index fingertip
- **Ulnar nerve:** fifth fingertip

Evaluation Format

The first purpose of an evaluation is to determine if a serious injury has occurred. The evaluation format of history, observation, palpation and special tests are thoroughly covered in Chapter 2 and Chapter 6. Listed below is an abbreviated version of this format.

(H) History
Questions should include mechanism of injury, location of pain, sensations experienced, and previous injury.

(O) Observation
Compare the uninvolved to the involved upper extremity and look for bleeding, deformity, swelling, discoloration, scars, and other signs of trauma.

(P) Palpation
Using bilateral comparison, palpate neurological, circulatory, and anatomical structures, and assess for potential fractures.

(S) Special Tests
Special tests assess disability to ligament, muscle, tendon, accessory anatomical structures, inflammatory conditions, range of motion, and pain or weakness in the affected area. These tests should be performed by a qualified allied health professional.

Assessment Tests

All injured joints should be properly evaluated. The purpose of a thorough evaluation is to enable the allied health professional to properly assess the severity of the injury and to make recommendations regarding treatment and possible return to participation. Listed below is a review of evaluation techniques utilized by certified athletic trainers. For further information, the learner should consult this chapter's references for a comprehensive description of assessment tests.

Elbow

Tests for Ligament Stability
- Valgus or abduction stress: evaluates the medial (ulna) collateral ligament stability of the elbow
- Varus or adduction stress: evaluates the lateral (radial) collateral ligament stability of the elbow

Epicondylitis Tests—Lateral
- Resisted wrist extension: determines the presence of lateral epicondylitis
- Resisted long finger extension: determines the presence of lateral epicondylitis
- Palmar flexion-pronation stretch: determines the presence of lateral epicondylitis

Epicondylitis Tests—Medial
- Resisted wrist flexion: determines the presence of medial epicondylitis
- Wrist extension-supination stretch: determines the presence of medial epicondylitis

Neurological Dysfunction Tests
- Tinel's sign—elbow: detects inflammation or entrapment of the ulnar nerve pronator teres syndrome: detects inflammation or entrapment of the median nerve
- Pinch grip: detects anterior interosseous nerve dysfunction

Wrist and Hand

Bony integrity tests
- Anatomical snuffbox compression: indicates possibility of a scaphoid (navicular) fracture
- Murphy's sign: test for dislocation of the lunate

Ligamentous Tests (fingers/thumb)
- PIP and DIP collateral ligament: assesses the stability of the radial and ulna ligaments of the phalanges
- MCP collateral ligament: assesses the stability of the radial and ulna ligaments of the metacarpophalangeal joints
- Gamekeeper's thumb: assesses the ulnar collateral ligament stability at the metacarpophalangeal joint

Musculoskeletal Tests
- Finkelstein's: determines presence of tenosynovitis in the abductor pollicis longus and extensor pollicis brevis tendons of the thumb (de Quervain's syndrome)
- Flexor digitorum superficialis: assesses flexor digitorum superficialis tendon function
- Flexor digitorum profundus: assesses flexor digitorum profundus tendon function
- Mallet finger: assesses extensor tendon integrity at the DIP joint
- Boutonniere deformity: assesses central slip integrity of extensor tendon at PIP joint

Carpal Tunnel Tests
- Phalen's or wrist press: detects presence of carpal tunnel syndrome
- Tinel's sign—wrist: detects presence of carpal tunnel syndrome

Conditions that Indicate an Athlete Should be Referred for Physician Evaluation

- Suspected fracture or dislocation
- Significant pain, especially on joint movement
- Circulation or neurological impairment
- Joint instability
- Loss of sensation (motor or sensory)
- Abnormal sensations such as clicking, popping, grating or weakness
- Any doubt about severity or nature of the injury

Common Injuries

Sprain

Injuries to the elbow, forearm, wrist, and hand joints are common. With a mechanism of excessive stress to the joint, injuries to ligaments are classified as sprains. Sprains are placed into one of three categories: first degree (mild), second degree (moderate), or third degree (severe).

First degree sprain. One or more of the supporting ligaments and surrounding tissues are stretched. There is minor discomfort, point tenderness, and little or no swelling. There is no abnormal movement in the joint to indicate lack of stability.

Second degree sprain. A portion of one or more ligaments is torn. There is pain, swelling, point tenderness, and loss of function for several minutes or longer. There is slight abnormal movement in the joint. The athlete may not be able to move extremity. Additionally, an accompanying fracture is possible in all degrees of sprain.

Third degree sprain. One or more ligaments have been completely torn, resulting in joint instability. There is either extreme pain or little pain (if nerve damage has occurred), loss of function, point tenderness, and rapid swelling. An accompanying avulsive fracture is possible.

As with any injury, the basic treatment of protection, rest, ice, compression, elevation, and support (PRICES), along with medical referral should be utilized.

Olecranon Bursitis

Inflammation by either direct blow (contusion) or overuse will cause inflammation of the olecranon bursa. Inflammation to the bursa results in the affected area having a thick and warm feeling. When this occurs, referral to a physician is essential. Once this condition has been evaluated, basic treatment could include ice or heat, and external compression (elastic wrap).

Carpal Tunnel Syndrome

This medical condition is caused by pressure on the median nerve. Symptoms occur as a result from constriction in the carpal tunnel and pressure on the median nerve. Treatment of carpal tunnel syndrome usually begins with a wrist splint, rest and medications. Non-surgical treatments help temporarily in many cases, especially if symptoms are mild. If unsuccessful, medical re-evaluation is recommended.

Scaphoid Fracture

One of the most disabling conditions in sports, a fracture to the scaphoid (navicular) is common. Since these injuries usually result from a fall on an extended wrist, fractured navicular bone often leads to non-union of the bone fragments due to its poor blood supply. Usually severe pain is located in the anatomical snuffbox. Medical treatment requires PRICES, X-ray, and re-evaluation on a weekly basis.

Dislocation/Subluxation

Injuries to the head of the radius, lunate, and phalanges (fingers) are common sites of dislocations and subluxations. Most of these injuries occur from force placed on an outstretched hand with the elbow in extension. Some of these dislocations are obvious to recognize while some are not. For example, some of the various types of wrist dislocations (lunate, perilunate, transscaphoid-perilunate) can be easily missed. Therefore careful and through evaluation should be performed and proper referral if there is a suspicion of abnormal joint alignment or function. As with all dislocations, always suspect a fracture. Medical referral for a comprehensive evaluation is needed.

Epicondylitis

A medical term with a suffix of "itis" means inflammation. Epicondylitis is classified as a inflammation of the epicondyle and the tissues adjoining the humerus. Common sites for epicondylitis is in the elbow joint. Medial (inside) epicondylitis is referred to as pitchers elbow, whereas tennis elbow affects the lateral (outside) epicondyle, pitcher (little league) elbow.

Contusion

These injuries are caused by a direct blow or by falling on the extremity. Contusion is a bruising of tissue, which commonly occurs to the hand and ulna side of the forearm. Basic first-aid treatment would be protection, rest, ice, compression, elevation, PRICES, and support.

Subungual Hematoma

When the fingernail receives a contusion (bruise), a subungual hematoma can occur. This excessive force will develop an accumulation of blood under the fingernail. Immediate treatment includes ice and medical referral to remove the fluid (blood).

Boxer's Fracture

A fracture of the metacarpal bone(s) of the hand at the neck of the metacarpal near the metacarpal head. A boxer's fracture usually occurs to the fifth and/or fourth metacarpal and is caused from striking a hard object/surface with a closed fist.

Bennett's Fracture

This is a fracture-dislocation of the base of first metacarpal of the hand. The unstable nature of this fracture results in the 1st metacarpal displacing into the carpometacarpal joint. Bennett fracture must be identified and referred acutely for proper treatment. This unstable fracture usually requires surgery to restore normal alignment and function.

Mallet Finger

A tendon rupture or avulsion of the extensor tendon at the distal interphalangeal joint of the finger. This is usually caused by a direct blow to the tip of the finger that rapidly/forcefully flexes the interphalangeal joint. If not identified and treated acutely, Mallet Finger will result in a permanent deformity to the finger.

Jersey Finger

A tendon rupture or avulsion of the flexor digitorum profundus at the distal interphalangeal joint. This is commonly caused by the classic "jersey tackle." The finger firmly grips the jersey in flexion but is forced/pulled in extension as the jersey is ripped from the grasp. This injury occurs most commonly to the ring (fourth) finger but can occur to any of the fingers. Jersey finger must be identified and treated acutely (usually surgically) to restore normal finger function.

Throwing Injuries to the Elbow

Overhead throwing injuries to the elbow are very common in variety of sports (baseball, softball, volleyball, javelin, tennis, etc.). Overhead throwing is a high-speed, highly ballistic activity that requires careful management and well-thought-out preparation. Some of the pathologies that can occur due to overhead throwing include medial epicondylitis, medial (ulna) collateral ligament sprain or rupture, tendinopathy, bone spurs, ulnar nerve injury, and growth plate injuries in children. Many of these pathologies are classified as overuse injuries and once present must be treated with rest and rehabilitation. Prevention is a key component for many of these pathologies. Some important factors in prevention of overhead throwing injures are as follows:

- Warm up to throw (don't use throwing as a warm-up exercise)
- Implement sport-specific strengthening exercises for forearm flexor/pronator muscle group
- Teach proper throwing mechanics
- Implement a progressive throwing program (progression over time of velocity, distance, and number of throws)
- Get in throwing shape before throwing competitively
- Restrict high pitch counts
- No "trick pitches" (curveball, slider) before physically mature
- Allow proper rest/recovery (avoid throwing on short rest)
- Don't throw with pain

Musculoskeletal Conditions/Disorders

Listed next are musculoskeletal conditions/disorders that affect the elbow, wrist, and/or hand. Define and review these conditions using a medical dictionary.

Elbow and Forearm
- Elbow hyperextension
- Forearm splints
- Ganglion
- Nerve injury (median, radial, ulnar)
- Osteochondritis dissecans
- Supracondylar fracture
- Volkman's fracture
- Volkmann's dschemic contracture

Wrist and Hand
- Barton fracture
- Baseball finger
- Bennett fracture
- Boutonniere deformity
- Boxers fracture
- Colles' fracture
- Felon
- Gamekeeper's thumb
- Mallet finger

- Murphy's sign
- Profundus tendon rupture (Jersey finger)
- Smith's fracture

Rehabilitation

Sending an athlete back to competition before healing is complete leaves the player susceptible to further injury. The best way to determine when healing is complete is by the absence of pain during stressful activity and by the return of full range of motion and strength, power and endurance to the affected muscle group. Prior to the beginning of any rehabilitation exercise program, the certified athletic trainer should consult with the sports medicine team to establish an individual program tailored for that individual athlete and the specific injury to be rehabilitated. The following list of exercises can be used as rehabilitative or preventive exercises.

Range of Motion Exercises
- Elbow
- Flexion
- Extension
- Supination
- Pronation

Wrist
- Flexion
- Extension
- Radial deviation
- Ulnar deviation
- Supination
- Pronation

Fingers
- Flexion
- Extension
- Abduction
- Adduction
- Opposition

Resistance/Strengthening Exercises
Elbow
Arm flexion (bicep curls)
Arm extension (triceps extension)

Wrist, Hand, and Fingers
Hand squeeze
Finger abduction
Pinch grip
Lateral/key pinch grip

To view videos and other materials related to this chapter on the ELBOW, FOREARM, WRIST, AND HAND, see access instructions on the last page of this text.

Return to Competition Guidelines
Before returning to competition, the following rehabilitation guidelines must be met:
- Full range of motion
- Strength, power, and endurance are proportional to the athlete's size and sport
- No pain in upper extremity during running, jumping, or cutting

Preventive/Supportive Techniques

Whether to apply adhesive and/or elastic bandages to an uninjured anatomical structure is a decision the certified athletic trainer will have to make. All injured joints should be supported initially. The basic taping and wrapping techniques are listed.

Wrapping Techniques for Compression
Elbow compression wrap
Wrist/hand compression wrap

Taping Techniques for the Elbow
Elbow hyperextension elbow
Epicondylitis

Taping Techniques for the Forearm, Wrist, and Hand
Forearm splint
Wrist
Thumb spica
Thumb C-lock
Finger splint
Collateral interphalangeal joint
Hyperextension of phalanges
Contusion to hand

Protective Devices

The use of protective devices is beneficial, if they are properly selected, used in the appropriate setting, correctly fitted, properly applied, and used within the rules and guidelines of the specific sport. Consultation with an equipment specialist and certified athletic trainer is highly encouraged. Listed next are various protective devices that are commercially available to use as an adjunct or replacement to a taping or wrapping procedures.
- Archery forearm protectors
- Counter force forearm band
- Elbow pads counter force forearm band
- Elbow hyperextension brace
- Elbow pads
- Forearm pads
- Hand pads
- Hyperextension braces
- Lateral/medial elbow strap
- Olecranon pad
- Specialized gloves
- Wrist braces
- Wrist hyperextension braces

Elbow Compression Wrap

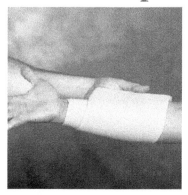 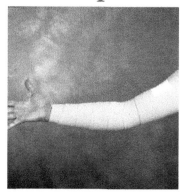

1. Begin the 6" elastic wrap at the wrist, spiral the wrap around the forearm and above the elbow joint.
2. Secure the wrap with a small strip of 1 1/2" adhesive tape.

Wrist/Hand Compression Wrap

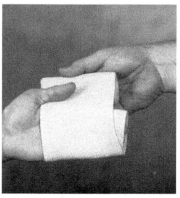 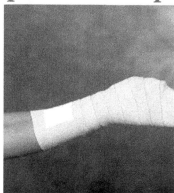

1. Begin the 4" elastic wrap at the finger tips, spiral around the hand and above the wrist.
2. Secure the wrap with a small strip of 1-1/2" adhesive tape.

Elbow Hyperextension

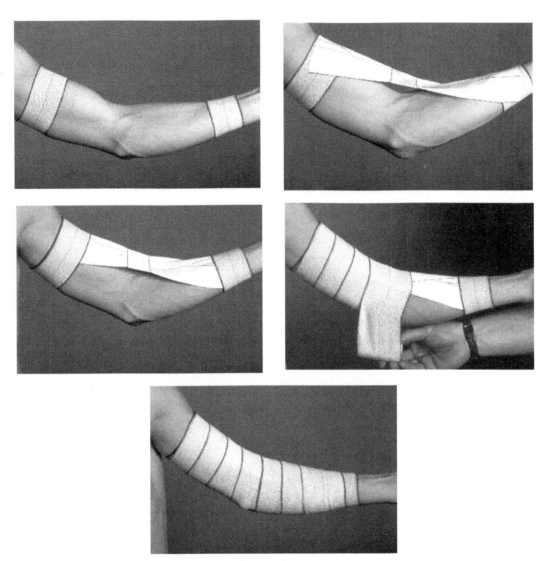

1. Apply two anchor strips of 2" elastic tape. The proximal anchor will be positioned above the belly of the biceps muscle and the distal anchor will be positioned on the distal one-third of the forearm.
2. Using 1 1/2" adhesive tape, construct a five to seven strip butterfly. Prior to application, place a strip of tape around the mid portion of this support pattern. Apply the butterfly pattern from the proximal anchor to the distal anchor. Apply proper tension to insure that the elbow does not reach full extension.
3. A second series of anchor strips should be applied, using elastic tape.
4. A final continuous closure strip is applied with 2" elastic tape. Begin on the distal anchor and spiral the tape, overlapping one-half its width, and ending on the proximal anchor.

Wrist

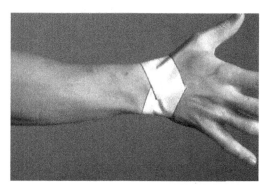 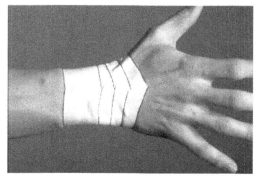

Technique A: In certain sporting activities, tape should not be applied to the palm of the hand. In such situations, apply two layers of four support strips. Begin proximally and work distally. Apply the 1-1/2" adhesive tape around the wrist starting at the ulnar condyle, cross the dorsal aspect of the distal forearm, and encircle the wrist. Overlap the tape by one-half its width each time. The second layer should be applied proximally to distally and should cover the same area.

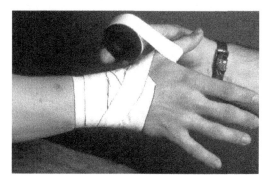 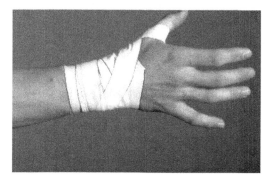

Technique B: In conjunction with Technique A, include a thumb spica taping procedure. Starting at the ulnar condyle, cross the dorsum of the hand, cover the lateral joint line, encircle the thumb, proceed across the palmar aspect of the hand, and finish at the ulnar condyle.

Thumb Spica

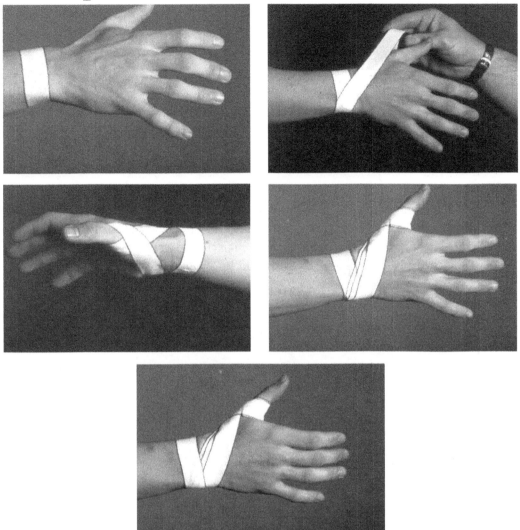

1. Apply an anchor strip of adhesive tape around the wrist. Start at the ulnar condyle, cross the dorsal aspect of the distal forearm, and encircle the wrist.
2. Apply the first of three support strips for the first MP joint. Starting at the ulnar condyle, cross the dorsum of the hand, cover the lateral joint line, encircle the thumb, proceed across the palmar aspect of the hand, and finish at the ulnar condyle.
3. This is commonly referred to as a thumb spica. Repeat this procedure.
4. To help hold this procedure in place, apply a final anchor strip around the wrist. Check for circulation/skin color at the distal phalanx once the tape procedure is complete.

Adjunct Taping Procedures: Thumb Spica
These adjunct taping procedures can be used in conjunction with the basic technique presented.

Technique A: In another application of the thumb spica, tape is applied in the opposite direction.

Thumb C-Lock

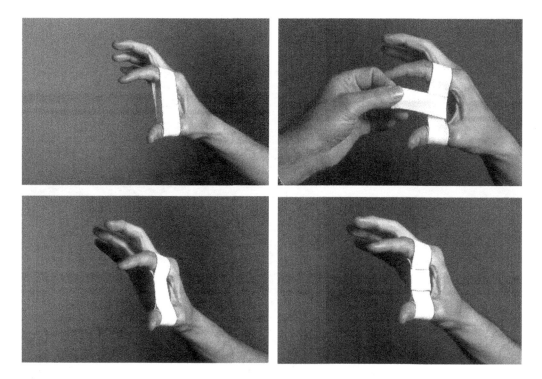

1. Apply a continuous strip of tape encircling the proximal aspects of the 1st and 2nd phalanges.
2. Between these phalanges, press the tape together.
3. To secure this technique, apply a strip of tape parallel to the first and second phalanges, that encircles the tape in the space between the thumb and index finger. This procedure restricts the thumb in abduction and extension. This procedure restricts the thumb in abduction and extension. Therefore, it is sometimes referred to as the butterfly, buddy taping, or check rein.

Contusion to Hand

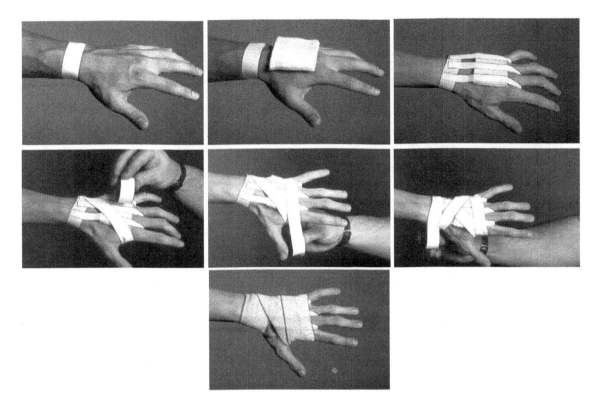

1. Apply an anchor strip of 1" adhesive tape around the wrist. Start at the ulnar condyle, cross the dorsal aspect of the distal forearm, and encircle the wrist.
2. The foam pad is then applied over the affected area of the hand.
3. Apply strips of 1/2" tape. Start on the palmar aspect of the anchor strip, cross between the phalanges, and end on the dorsal aspect of the anchor strip.
4. Three strips are applied, between the second and third, third and fourth, and fourth and fifth phalanges.
5. Next, apply a strip of 1" adhesive tape in a figure of eight pattern. Begin on wrist's dorsal aspect near the ulnar condyle, cross diagonally to the second metacarpal, encircling the distal aspect of the second through fifth metacarpals. Continue across the palmar aspect to the fifth metacarpal, crossing diagonally from here to the radial aspect of the wrist and encircle the wrist.
6. Two to three figure of eights can be applied. This technique is completed with a second anchor strip of 1" adhesive tape applied around the wrist.
7. A continuous figure of eight strip of 2" elastic tape is applied to give additional support.

References

Anderson, M., & Hall, S. (2012). *Foundations of athletic training* (5th ed.). Baltimore, MD: Lippincott Williams & Wilkins.

Andrews, J., Clancy, W., & Whiteside, J. (1997). *On-field evaluation and treatment of common athletic injuries.* St. Louis, MO: McGraw-Hill Higher Education.

Barker, S., Wright, K., & Wright, V. (2007). *Sports injuries 3D* (3rd ed.). Gardner, KS: Cramer Products, Inc.

Booher, J., & Thibodeau, G. (2000). *Athletic injury assessment* (4th ed.). St. Louis, MO: McGraw-Hill Higher Education.

Gallaspy, J., & May, D. (1996). *Signs and symptoms of athletic injuries.* St. Louis, MO: McGraw-Hill Higher Education.

Hoppenfeld, S. (1976). *Physical examination of the spine and extremities.* New York, NY: Appleton-Century Crofts.

Knight, K. (2010). *Developing clinical proficiencies in athletic training* (4th ed.). Champaign, IL: Human Kinetics.

Magee, D. (2008). *Orthopedic physical assessment* (5th ed.). Philadelphia, PA: W. B. Sanders.

Mellion, M., Walsh, W., & Shelton, G. (1990). *The team physician's handbook.* Philadelphia, PA: Hanley and Belfus, Inc.

National Safety Council. (2007). *First aid taking action.* St. Louis, MO: McGraw-Hill Higher Education.

Pfeiffer, R., & Mangus, B. (2012). *Concepts of athletic training* (6th ed.). Boston, MA: Jones and Bartlett.

Prentice, W. (2014). *Arnheim's principles of athletic training* (15th ed.). St. Louis, MO: McGraw-Hill Higher Education.

Prentice, W. (2011). *Rehabilitation techniques in sports medicine and athletic training* (5th ed.). St. Louis, MO: McGraw-Hill.

Prentice, W. (2009). Therapeutic modalities in sports medicine (6th ed.). St. Louis, MO: McGraw-Hill Higher Education.

Starkey, C. (2013). *Athletic training and sports medicine: An integrated approach* (5th ed.). Boston, MA: Jones and Bartlett.

Starkey, C., & Ryan, J. (2010). *Evaluation of orthopedic and athletic injuries* (3th ed.). Philadelphia, PA: F. A. Davis.

Starkey, C. (2013). *Therapeutic modalities* (4th ed.). Philadelphia, PA: F. A. Davis.

Stedman's medical dictionary for the health professions and nursing (7th ed.). (2011). Baltimore, MD: Lippincott, Williams, & Wilkins.

Street, S., & Rumkle, D. (2000). *Athletic protective equipment: Care, selection, and fitting.* St. Louis, MO: McGraw-Hill Higher Education.

Taber's medical dictionary (22nd ed.). (2013). Philadelphia: F. A. Davis.

Thompson, C., & Floyd, R. (2012). *Manual of structural kinesiology* (18th ed.). St. Louis, MO: McGraw-Hill Higher Education.

Wright, K., Whitehill, W., & Lewis., M. (2005). *Preventive techniques: Taping/wrapping techniques and protective devices.* Gardner, KS: Cramer Products.

Suggested Multimedia Resources

Wright, K., & Whitehill, W. (1996). *Sports medicine taping series: The shoulder and elbow.* St. Louis, MO: McGraw-Hill Higher Education.

Wright, K., & Whitehill, W. (1996). *Sports medicine taping series: The wrist and hand.* St. Louis, MO: McGraw-Hill Higher Education.

Wright, K., Harrelson, G., Floyd, R., & Fincher, L. (1994). *Sports medicine evaluation series: The elbow.* St. Louis, MO: Mosby Year Book, Inc.

Wright, K., Harrelson, G., Floyd, R., & Fincher, L. (1994). *Sports medicine evaluation series: The wrist and hand.* St. Louis, MO: Mosby Year Book, Inc.

Review Questions

Completion

1. The_____and_____tests assess the elbow collateral ligaments.

2. The anatomical snuffbox test can help identify a possible of the scaphoid bone.

3. _____is the accumulation of blood under the fingernail.

4. Pronation and supination are suggested exercises for_____rehabilitation.

5. The bones that form the elbow are the_____,_____, and _____.

6. The _____is similar to the femur of the leg, as both have two_____at their_____or   lower ends.

7. Of the two bones of the forearm, the_____acts as a stationary axle.

8. The elbow joint has very strong_____and_____support.

9. Helping to stabilize the elbow joint, by attaching to the ulna and encircling the head of the radius, is the_____ligament.

10. The three muscles that control the movement of the elbow are the _____,_____, and the_____.

11. The wrist joint is formed by the distal ends of the_____and_____, and by the _____bones.

Short Answer

1. Name the three ligaments of the elbow joint.

2. List two suggested exercises for rehabilitation of the wrist and hand.

3. Name the eight bones that make up the wrist.

4. Name the three groups of bones of the hand.

13 Environmental and Other Important Issues to Consider in Athletic Health Care

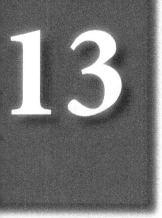

Educational Objectives

Upon completing this chapter, the reader will be able to do the following:
- Recognize the various environmental conditions that affect sport participants
- Recognize the signs and symptoms of nutritional disorders among athletes
- Identify time travel conditions and their adverse effect on human performance
- Identify common cold, respiratory tract infections, and medical illnesses in athletes
- Recognize use of performance enhancing drugs and their effects on sport participants

Environmental Conditions

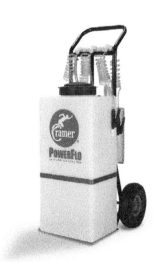

There are three basic environmental conditions that impact athletic performance: heat, cold, and altitude. All three can have a negative effect on performance. The athletic trainer, coach, and athlete must prepare for these conditions. The guidelines for prevention and symptoms of environmental distress are discussed in this chapter.

Heat-Related Conditions (Hyperthermia)

High temperatures and elevated humidity can negatively impact athletic performance, adversely affect health, and even threaten life. While environmental heat problems will occur in sport and one of the more important concepts to implement is to have a plan in place prior to the start of any season that addresses the issues of environmental issues that has been agreed upon by all parties (coaches, parents, administrators, and the health care providers).

Exercise generates heat that the body must dissipate. If the body retains too much heat, the victim can die. The body cools itself mainly through the sweating mechanism; heat is carried away from the body as perspiration evaporates. This cooling process can be interrupted in two ways: the humidity can be so high that sweat does not evaporate, or the thermoregulatory system of the athlete can be disrupted, causing sweating to cease. The coach and athletic training student can help prevent heat related problems in several ways described below.

1. Pre-hydration and Rehydration

Frequent fluid intake before, during, and after practice will help ensure that athletes function efficiently and safely. The weight an athlete loses through exertion is almost entirely related to fluid loss. A fluid loss of as little as 3% of total body weight can adversely affect endurance and coordination. Such fluid loss can initiate heat illness. There are several reasons for athletes to prehydrate. First, they need to replace lost fluid from the previous practice session. Second, thirst is not an accurate indicator of the need for fluid. A thirsty person will feel rehydrated well before the adequate intake of fluids. Third, drinking too much water at one time will give the athlete an uncomfortable feeling. Several smaller doses of water are better than one large amount. One strategy for replacing fluids is to drink cold water and 6% to 8% solutions of carbohydrate using the following formula:

Dehydration

the process of water loss by the body

> 34 oz. two hours before activity
> 13 - 17 oz. 15 minutes before activity
> 13 - 17 oz. every 30 minutes during activity

Additionally, body weight, exertion, and duration of exercise will have an impact on these recommended fluid intakes. During peak exertion, when gastric emptying is most crucial, it is better to provide athletes with water or electrolyte drinks with a carbohydrate concentration of 6% or less. It is best to use electrolyte drinks before and after practice, when gastric emptying time is less crucial.

> **DO NOT deny an athlete water or rest at ANY time.**

2. Acclimatization

While humans cannot adjust to being deprived of water, they can get better acclimated to hot weather. This process can take 1-2 weeks of working out in heat with gradually increased intensity.

Acclimatization

the process of getting the body used to the weather conditions for sport

3. Pre-participation Physical Examination

With all individuals receiving a medical evaluation, athletes should be asked about previous occurrence of heat illness problems. Identification of susceptible individuals should be noted and monitored.

4. Wear Proper Clothing

Light, loose fitting clothing will allow air to move over the body. Clothing that binds can trap heat. Helmets should be taken off during breaks. Do not allow athletes to work out in rubberized clothing or sweat suits in the false belief that they are accelerating weight loss. The weight loss will be easily replaced by fluid, not fat loss. Also, perspiration will be trapped, the cooling process will be interrupted, and the stage will be set for dehydration and heat illness.

5. Use Weight Charts

The athletic training student can weigh all same sex players before and after each practice. Athletes who do not regain their lost water weight by the start of the next practice should be encouraged to replace fluids. If there is significant fluid loss (3% or more of body weight), the team physician should be contacted. Be aware of athletes who may have disorders eating and a possible need to weight an athlete backward if weight is a triggering issue for them.

6. Monitor Environmental Conditions

It is advised to monitor the environmental conditions through local weather monitoring systems. High temperature and humidity will affect an athlete's ability to release body temperature and physical activity should be monitored on these days. There should be emphasis that a plan be in place and agreed upon by medical staff, coaching staff and administration regarding the intensity of practice permitted during high heat stress days. Establish rules prior to the need and follow the rules when appropriate.

7. Be Prepared to Give First Aid

Know the signs of heat exhaustion and heat stroke and be prepared to provide first aid.

8. Adequate Rest

Athletes need to have adequate periods of rest between athletic sessions and from day to day.

9. Diets High in Electrolytes

Provide nutritional education for athletes as it relates to diets high in replacement electrolytes and especially sodium. Fruits and vegetables (i.e. oranges, bananas, corn, green beans) are good sources of foods high in electrolytes. Normal salt use is encouraged in the diet of an athlete to meet electrolyte needs: table salt, pickles, ketchup, mustard, and canned foods such as soups are excellent ways to increase sodium normally in the diet.

10. Awareness of Ongoing Illnesses and/or Conditions

Athletes who are taking medicines and/or suffered from recent gastrointestinal distress are at a higher risk for heat related illness. It should be noted that athletes should keep the sports medicine staff and coaches informed of any pre-existing medical conditions (i.e. asthma, sickle cell trait, and any form of a prior heat related illness). Additionally, the medical staff and coaches should monitor these individuals in all types of physical activity.

Fluid Replacement

Dehydration, which is probably the primary cause of the heat illnesses listed below, can occur not only in hot humid weather, but also during the coldest days of the year. Athletes can lose 5 to 10 pounds of fluid weight during one hot, humid practice session. After practice, drink 12+ fluid ounces for each pound lost. Strenuous winter workouts in the gym can have the same effect. In addition, during the winter the body loses essential fluids in ways besides sweating. The air inside heated buildings and outdoors is almost always drier during the winter than in the summer. It must be warmed and moisturized before the lungs can absorb it. During this process, the body uses fluids and energy at a very rapid rate, calling for continuous fluid replacement. The body's thirst mechanism isn't always accurate, especially in the winter. Athletes may not feel as thirsty as they did on that hot summer afternoon, but may need as much fluid and electrolyte replacement as possible, preferably 4 to 8 ounces of fluid per every 20 minutes of exercise. Athletes need to continually hydrate during the day before practices or games. By being properly hydrated, it will help the athlete achieve their best performance and avoid heat illnesses caused by improper hydration. Remind athletes that if they wait until they are thirsty to drink, they are already becoming dehydrated.

Heat Cramps (Hyperthermia)

Heat cramps are the least serious of heat illnesses/hyperthermia. They are however, the first sign that the body may be having difficulty with increased temperature and a warning sign that more serious problems may soon develop if proper steps are not taken to cool and rehydrate the athlete. The most common sites for heat cramps are the lower extremities and abdominal cavity. Athletic trainers, coaches, and athletic training students should review heat illnesses with the team physician and certified athletic trainers before the start of the season so they will be prepared in the event of heat illnesses. Athletic trainers, coaches, and student athletic Ttrainers should look for any or all of the following signs if they suspect the athlete may be suffering from heat exhaustion.

Signs and Symptoms
- Profuse sweating
- Involuntary cramping of the muscles

First-Aid Procedures
- Moving the athlete to a cooler location
- Providing the athlete with cool fluids (water and/or electrolyte drinks)
- Instruct the athlete to stretch, apply ice and or massage the affected area
- Monitor the athlete for signs of other heat and/or illness problems

Heat Exhaustion (Hyperthermia)

Heat exhaustion

the process of overheating, that if cared for can be relieved without advanced medical care

Heat exhaustion is more serious and may be more difficult to recognize than heat cramps. However, it is usually not life threatening, but if not treated properly, it can become a medical emergency. This condition may be caused by many variables such as: athletes exposed to high temperatures for long periods, improper hydration, improper clothing, and/or lack of conditioning/acclimatization. Heat exhaustion begins when the thermoregulatory system of the body starts to fail. Athletic trainers, coaches, and athletic training students should look for any or all of the following signs and/or symptoms if they suspect the athlete may be suffering from heat exhaustion.

Signs and Symptoms
- Cool, moist, or pale skin color
- Headache, lightheadedness, dizziness, lack of coordination
- Profuse sweating, decreased urine output, diarrhea
- Fast and shallow breathing
- Weak but rapid pulse (less than 120 beats per minute)
- Dilated pupils
- Nausea/vomiting
- Muscle cramps
- General sense of weakness /tiredness
- Conscious, but fainting may occur
- Watch for signs of shock

First-Aid Procedures
- Immediately remove the athlete from direct sunlight if possible
- Remove excessive clothing and equipment
- Assess vital signs
- Start reducing the athlete's temperature immediately.
- Cool the body with ice towels, ice bags on neck, head, armpits, and groin.
- Place the athlete in a recumbent position.
- Encourage the athlete to drink cool fluids such as water or electrolyte drinks.
- Athletes should gradually progress to full participation under close observation.

Heat Stroke (Hyperthermia)

Heat stroke

the most extreme form of overheating, a medical emergency

Heat stroke is the most serious form of hyperthermia; it is a life-threatening medical emergency! Athletes who reach this stage of heat illnesses usually have a high body temperature (104 degree F or higher), are dehydrated, and usually have some form of electrolyte imbalance. The body's thermoregulatory system begins to fail and the brain is no longer able to send messages to the rest of the body telling it how to cool off. In essence, the body is sending too much blood to the surface of the skin in an attempt to cool itself down. By doing this, blood is being diverted rapidly away from the internal organs, which in turn begin to shut down. This may result in the athlete going into a coma or even death. Athletic trainers, coaches, and athletic training students should look for any or all of the following signs and/or symptoms if they suspect the athlete may be suffering from heat stroke:

Signs and Symptoms
- Skin is hot, dry, red
- Athlete is mentally confused and may be very aggressive
- Elevated temperature
- Headache/dizzy, weak and fatigued feeling
- Possible absence of sweating
- Strong, rapid pulse (>160)
- Falling blood pressure
- Elevated core temp (104 degree F or higher)
- Convulsions
- Conscious but unresponsive aphasic
- Diarrhea/vomiting
- Athlete may faint or become unconscious

First-Aid Procedures
- Activate EMS–911 immediately.
- Remove excessive clothing and equipment, move out of direct sunlight and into air conditioning immediately if possible.
- Check vital signs.
- Cool athlete as quickly as possible (cold bath immersion, ice towels, ice bags on neck, head, armpits, and groin).
- If the athlete is conscious and responsive, give cold fluids.
- Athletes MUST be cleared by a physician before returning to sports activities and gradually progress from limited participation to full participation over several days under close observation for a return of symptoms.

While heat exhaustion is more common than heat stroke, the later is much more serious. Therefore, transportation to advanced medical care is a top priority and cooling of the body must be started immediately. The functions of the central nervous system will be impaired and educational information on heat stress can be found at Centers for Disease Control and Prevention website, www.cdc.gov/niosh/topics/heatstress

Cold Weather Conditions

Frostbite

In severely cold conditions, frostbite becomes another major concern for athletes. Late-autumn football games are sometimes played in subfreezing air temperatures. When combined with wind, these low temperatures can freeze unprotected skin tissue. The most susceptible areas are the fingers, toes, ears, and exposed parts of the face. Common frostbite warning signals include a tingling or burning sensation, pain, numbness, and discoloration of the skin (frostbitten areas have a yellow-white, waxy appearance). In extreme cold, however, flesh may freeze quickly, without warning, due to the cold's anesthetizing effect on the skin. Keeping cold and dampness away from the skin is the best protection against frostbite. You can also help ward off frostbite with physical actions, such as wiggling fingers and toes, making faces, and working the muscles to increase the supply of blood to various areas. If frostbite should occur, medical referral is recommended. Be sure to notify your athletic trainer if you suspect that an athlete is suffering from frostbite.

Hypothermia

Any athlete who participates in outdoor recreation should guard against excessive heat loss and recognize the following progressive signs of hypothermia, a potentially fatal condition. Those signs include the following:

- Constant shivering; this is an attempt by the body to generate heat
- Apathy, slurring of speech, listlessness, involuntary muscle movement, croaky voice, sleepiness, and generalized rigidity of muscles
- Sluggishness or clumsiness, poor judgment
- Unconsciousness, pupils that are abnormally dilated and that react sluggishly to light, and very slow pulse and respiratory rates
- Freezing of hands and/or feet
- Athletes with asthma (make sure you store their asthma inhalers so medication remains at normal temperature, avoiding adverse reactions)

If nothing is done to prevent further loss of body heat or to start the warming process once these stages have begun, hypothermia can be fatal. For this reason, prompt initial care is of utmost importance. If you suspect that an athlete is suffering from hypothermia, take the athlete to a warm area, remove any wet clothing and gradually warm the body in warm, dry blankets. Immediately notify emergency personnel as well as your athletic trainer.

Altitude

The third type of environmental condition that can be experienced by athletes is altitude. When an athlete trains at one altitude level and then must compete at another altitude level, these athletes can experience an impact on their performances. Typically the negative impact occurs when an athlete who has trained at a low altitude level must compete at a significantly higher altitude level. This impacts performance because the higher altitude has less oxygen concentration. This makes it more difficult for the athlete to supply the required amount of oxygen to the body's systems. This negative impact is usually seen with sports that are aerobic in nature. Anaerobic sporting events result in less of an impact because the event is over before the body experiences an oxygen debt. To avoid this condition, athletes should be given the opportunity to train at the higher elevations for a period of time that allows their bodies to adjust to the limited oxygen atmosphere.

Nutrition

What and when an athlete eats can affect performance. Common advice is that an individual should wait an hour or more after eating to exercise pending composition of food choice. Although athletes with full stomachs will not necessarily have performance problems, there is some truth in this advice. It is a fact that when there is food in the stomach, more blood is required for digestion and that during physical activity, the active muscles need more blood. Therefore, unless an adequate amount of blood can be pumped out in order to fulfill both needs, either the digestion process or the working muscles will be in short supply of blood. This can cause stomach cramping, other digestive upsets, and overall muscle weakness.

Athletes vary in their ability to exercise after eating (or without eating). Some complain of becoming dizzy or weak during practice unless they have a snack beforehand. Eating a substantial, well-balanced meal can help prevent dizziness or weakness during activity. Normal gastric emptying (from the stomach into the small intestine) can take from one to four hours, depending on the composition of the meal. High carbohydrate and liquid meals will pass through the digestive system more quickly than meals high in fats and proteins. Another factor in digestion rate is how well food is chewed. The stomach has to work harder on food that hasn't been adequately chewed, and it holds it for a longer period of time. This often causes a feeling of fullness or bloating.

If an athlete eats an ideal pre-competition meal and still experiences hunger pangs or weakness during and after practice, they may need an extra snack, as long as the feeling of having food in the stomach does not interfere with their athletic performance. However, they should select small portions of foods that are not spicy or bulky and that are easily digested. Pre-activity foods should exclude the following items:

- Fatty foods, because they are digested slowly and can interfere with efficiency in exercise
- Gas-forming foods, such as bulky raw vegetables, that can cause discomfort and detract from physical abilities
- Salt tablets (average diet usually contains enough salt)
- Special "magic" foods (such as energy drinks)
- Nutritional supplements can be costly and potentially dangerous, possibly containing stimulants.

A wise selection for pre- and post-activity eating is a menu that is low in fat content, nongaseous, nonalcoholic, well balanced, and high in carbohydrates. A good example would be a meal that includes broiled chicken, a baked potato, green beans, skim milk, and a baked apple. To replace diminished glycogen stores, post-exercise menus should also emphasize carbohydrate-rich foods. Fluid replacement should include two cups (16 oz.) of liquid for every pound lost and drink until urine is light colored or "lemonade" colored. Suggest to athletes that they avoid consuming beverages containing caffeine, such as soft drinks, tea, and coffee, before practices and games. Beverages containing caffeine stimulate the flow of urine, which may cause discomfort during competition or decrease the body's water level before competition, adversely affecting performance. Instead, athletes should drink plenty of plain water or electrolyte drinks to ensure that they are well hydrated before practices and games. Remember that the total diet consumed during the days before the event is far more important than the meal eaten immediately prior to strenuous exercise.

Eating Disorders

Society has placed an emphasis on these issues in the last 30 years through the media images. Disordered eating affects females primarily, but male athletes are also frequently affected, especially in the sports that have weight classifications.

Anorexia Nervosa

A person refusing to eat or not eating enough to maintain normal body functions such as 15% below ideal body weight and loss of menses characterizes this disorder. This is commonly seen in the sports that have a high body image profile. Although the disorder can occur with any athlete, the sports most affected include, but are not limited to, cheerleading, gymnastics, cross country, swimming, wrestling, figure skating, and other sports that have weight classifications or weight limitations.

Bulimia

Overeating (binge) and then vomiting (purge) at least two times per week for three months characterizes this particular disorder. The athlete will consume large quantities of food and immediately purge the food through vomiting, laxatives, diet pills, or overexercise. This routine by the athlete is an attempt to gain essential energy requirements, but not the weight associated with the food. A person qualified in psychological disorders can best handle this psychological problem. The best plan of action by the athletic trainer is to refer the athlete to the most qualified health care provider. Helping the athlete develop a treatment plan that includes a psychologist, physician, and sports dietitian is key.

Female Athlete Triad

With the increase in participation among females in competitive sports in the last 25 years, there has been an increase in gender specific conditions. One such condition is the female athlete triad. This gender specific condition involves components of disorder eating, the absence of menstruation (amenorrhea), and loss of bone density (osteoporosis). The three separate conditions combine to give rise to this very serious and long-term disorder referred to as the female triad. When a female exhibits the signs associated with disordered eating, prompt referral is recommended.

Food and Vitamin Supplements

While food is important for both general health and athletic performance, the nutritional needs of athletes are only mildly different from those of their nonathletic peers. Misinformation concerning the role of nutrition and athletics can be confusing to the coach and athlete, sometimes leading to the improper and unnecessary use of food and vitamin supplements. One supplement that has received much medial attention is ephedra, a dangerous stimulant, which is now banned by the federal government. There are no "super foods" or wonder diets, and following dietary plans based on these concepts can result in an unbalanced diet and may actually interfere with peak athletic performance.

Supplement

a group of compounds that are not highly regulated by the U.S. Food and Drug Administration

Besides being an unnecessary expense, mega doses of vitamin supplements taken inappropriately can also lead to nutritional imbalances and can endanger the athlete's health. A balanced diet is the best way to give the body pep and energy. Thus, athletes should follow a nutritious diet that emphasizes a variety of high-carbohydrate, low fat foods. Since dietary supplements are not regulated by the Food and Drug Administration (FDA), athletes should not be encouraged to use items. These dietary supplements could be contaminated, harmful to their health, and/or banned by sport federations and anti-doping agencies. The following are on the NCAA nonpermissible sport food/supplements:

- Amino acids, including BCAAs
- Creatine
- Ginseng
- HMB
- Protein powders
- Taurine
- Nitrous oxide

Time Travel Conditions (Jet Lag)

One additional condition that can impact athletes is circadian dysrhythmia. This is when the body's internal clock is confused. This occurs when athletes travel across numerous time zones and is typically seen when the athlete travels from the west to the east. Both the eating and sleeping rhythms are disrupted and the athlete's internal clock is trying to adjust, but is having difficulty because of the day/night sequence. One important thing to remember is to keep your athletes well hydrated and limit caffeine.

Common Cold and Respiratory Tract Infections

Colds and other respiratory tract infections are common among athletes and can sideline an entire team if proper precautions are not taken. Contrary to what many believe, colds are primarily transmitted by touch, not by coughing and sneezing. These viruses are able to live for several days on hard surfaces, such as doorknobs, countertops, and equipment. All an athlete has to do to become infected is touch an infected surface and then transfer the virus to the respiratory system by rubbing the eyes or nose or touching the mouth. As a student athletic trainer, you should remind athletes to be especially conscious about keeping their hands clean and keeping them away from the eyes and nose. Also, avoid the use of a community towel or drinking cup, as viruses can live on them as well. Once an athlete has contracted a cold, there is no magic cure. Rest and light eating will generally be all that is necessary in treating the virus. As advised by their physician, nonprescription medication (aspirin or nonaspirin pain relievers) can minimize aching and discomfort by lowering fever. However, the physician may prescribe prescription medication to aid in recovery. For the Centers for Disease Control and Prevention recommendations on the use of antibiotics, please review the Antibiotics Aren't Always the Answer website at www.cdc.gov/Features/GetSmart/. However, as an athletic training student, you are not the one who should dispense these medications. Prior to return to activity, the athlete should be given adequate time to recover from the common cold or respiratory tract infection. Returning too soon can cause the virus to linger and possibly turn into a more serious illness.

Common Medical Conditions/Illnesses

In addition to skin conditions, the certified athletic trainer will be expected to evaluate for medical referral a number of medical illnesses. Once again, the range on these illnesses will be from mild to severe. The certified athletic trainer should realize his/her individual limitations and refer to the most appropriate health care provider when there is doubt as to the condition or treatment.

Amenorrhea
Cessation of the menstrual cycle and can be primary (never starting) or secondary (start and then stop for no reason). Often seen in athletes (cross country runners, gymnasts, or swimmers) due to training, diet, stress, and pregnancy.

Asthma
One of the most common conditions found in respiratory diseases is bronchial asthma. The causes are many and might include viral infections, stress, inhalation of bacteria, or changes in environmental conditions. Basically, bronchial asthma is characterized by a narrowing of the breathing passages, thus reducing the breathing of the affected individual. The best prevention is to identify those susceptible individuals and have them under the care of a physician and appropriate medication available to them. In sport, a specific type of asthma is EIA or exercised induced asthma. This is usually brought on in an asthmatic individual when they exercise.

Blister (Bullae)
A bleb or vesicle containing fluid (serum, blood, pus) sometimes caused by pressure; a collection of fluid below the epidermis.

Burn
Tissue injury resulting from excessive exposure to thermal, chemical, electrical, or radioactive agents. Classified in three categories:

- **First degree.** Superficial, damage limited to outer layer of the epidermis. Characterized by erythema, hyperemia, tenderness, and pain.
- **Second degree.** Damage extends through the epidermis and into the dermis, but not of sufficient extent to interfere with regeneration of epidermis. Vesicles present.
- **Third degree.** Both the epidermis and dermis are destroyed with damage extending into the underlying tissues. Tissue may be charred or coagulated.

Dysmenorrhea
Painful or difficult menstruation.
- **Primary.** Beginning with first period. No known etiology.
- **Secondary.** Originally normal, changed due to pathologic state.

Epilepsy
Recurrent disturbances of brain function that may be manifested as seizures, loss of consciousness, or psychic disturbances.

Hypertension (High Blood Pressure)
Sustained elevated blood pressure, systolic above 140, diastolic above 90 in adults.

Hyperventilation
Increased inspiration and expiration of air as a result of increase in rate or depth of respiration or both. Leads to decreased CO_2, increased O_2, respiratory alkalosis. Characterized by shortness of breath, lightheadedness, and perioral numbness.

Shock
A state of collapse resulting from acute peripheral circulatory failure. Characterized by blood pressure less than 90/60. May be caused by decreased volume and/or vasodilatation. Shock is a medical emergency!

Sunburn
Dermatitis due to exposure to the actinic (ultraviolet) rays of the sun.

Performance-Enhancing Drugs and Methods

The increased use of recreational drugs, prohibited substance, and prohibited methods by interscholastic, intercollegiate, amateur, and professional athletes has been recently exposed in the media and sport organizations. This has led to another area of great concern, the abuse of chemical agents by the very young athlete. Besides possibly starting such an athlete down a road of chemical dependency, drug and adverse use can have serious and sometimes irreversible side effects. For a more in-depth perspective on this subject, view the educational information offered by the Centers for Disease Control and Prevention (www.cdc.gov), Drug Free Sport (www.drugfreesport.com), and United States Anti-Doping Agency (USADA) www.usantidoping.org.

Marijuana
Marijuana is the second most commonly abused substance by the young athlete. The athletes who use marijuana, even on a casual basis, experience very significant effects that have a direct bearing on athletic performance. These effects include the following:
- Inhibition of the sweating mechanism in hot environments, which can lead to heat illness
- Major impairment of coordination as measured by hand steadiness, body sway, and accuracy of execution of movement
- Impairment of tracking performance, perceptual tasks, and vigilance

- Slowed reaction time to visual and auditory stimuli
- Altered perception of speed, time, and space
- Short-term and long-term memory loss
- Prolonged learning time

Probably the most serious effect of marijuana on the very young athlete is the establishment of a characteristic set of personality changes seen in marijuana users. This "anti-motivational syndrome" is characterized by apathy, loss of ambition and effectiveness, diminished ability to carry out long-term plans, difficulty in concentrating, decline in academic and athletic performance, intermittent confusion, impaired memory, and loss of energy.

Anabolic Steroids

Anabolic steroids, synthetic derivatives of the male hormone testosterone, are some of the most controversial drugs linked to athletics. Athletes hope to increase their strength and the size of their muscles through anabolic steroid use. Commonly, athletes on steroids also feel more aggressive and self-confident, which encourages them to train harder. There have been additional claims that steroids will do everything from increase red blood cell counts to act as glycogen-sparing (or energy-sparing) agents. The problem is that there is little conclusive evidence concerning the benefits of steroid use. Researchers agree that when normal, healthy men take steroids without training, there is no effect on muscle size or strength. The harmful side effects of steroid use have been much better documented than any strength gains. Among the side effects in males are liver damage (including liver cancer), impaired kidney function, enlargement of the prostate gland, decreased levels of natural testosterone, testicular atrophy resulting in sterility, growth of breast tissue, premature closure of epiphyseal plates in younger age groups, and weight gain caused by fluid retention which often leads to elevated blood pressure. Some of these side effects can even lead to death. In addition, the majority of athletes using steroids experience an increase in libido and detrimental aggressive behavior. In women, steroids can produce a deepened voice, growth of facial and chest hair, liver damage, clitoral enlargement, menstrual irregularities, and impairment of reproductive capacity. While the use of steroids have a negative effect on the cardiovascular system, recent research indicates that it also impact the levels of cholesterol, which over time has a very harmful effect on the body.

Alcohol

This is the most commonly abused drug at all levels. The peer pressure to drink is extreme. Because of its universal acceptance in our society, alcohol remains the most difficult drug to control. Alcohol, even taken after the contest, ultimately results in deterioration of the psychomotor skills of reaction time, eye-hand coordination, accuracy, balance, and complex coordination. Alcohol also impairs body temperature regulation, especially during prolonged exercise in cold environments. In addition, alcohol consistently decreases strength, power, local muscular endurance, speed, and cardiovascular endurance. Even though the athlete generally consumes alcohol in an attempt to gain psychological benefits, the psychomotor performance deteriorates first and most profoundly.

Tobacco Products

Recently, national sport governing bodies have taken the position that tobacco products are detrimental to the athlete and to the sport. Therefore, all persons associated with athletic participation have enacted rules and regulations to curb the use of tobacco products. Those tobacco products that have been identified as having a negative impact on the health of the athlete include all smoking, chewing, and snuff tobacco products. Case studies have shown that cancer is linked to the use of these products. The sport of baseball has seen the most recent regulations enacted to control the use of these products while at practice and in game situations. For additional information on prevention and cessation, visit www.cdc.gov/tobacco.

Caffeine

Moderate amounts of caffeine can increase mental alertness, but too much may cause anxiety, hamper performance, and increase heart rate. In endurance events lasting more than two hours, caffeine can enhance performance as it allows the body to burn more fatty acids as fuel. In addition, beverages containing caffeine have a diuretic effect. They stimulate the flow of urine, which may cause discomfort during activity or decrease the body's water level before competition, adversely affecting performance. IF an athlete insists on having caffeine, encourage moderation (one to two cups per day) with adequate hydration.

Dietary Supplements

The use of vitamins, minerals herbs, amino acids, proteins, energy products, and other dietary supplements can be questioned unless prescribed by the athletes' physician or other licensed healthcare provider. Since the federal government does not control and regulate the dietary supplement industry, athletes sometimes assume that everything is maintained at the high standards as controlled drugs. If questions arise, consult your physician or other licensed healthcare provider about their recommendations before taking dietary supplements. Adverse health issues along with positive drug test could result, which could affect athlete eligibility for further participation. For a more in-depth perspective on nutrition, view the CDC informational website at www.cdc.gov/nutrition/.

Recognition of Drug Use

Attempting to single out an individual as a user of recreational drugs, prohibited substance, and prohibited methods is a bias view and should be avoided. However, some of the individual changes may be seen in an athlete using drugs resemble the symptoms of severe personal or emotional problems. It is imperative to treat the athlete as an individual and to talk to him or her privately about the nature of the problem.

Signs of drug use include the following:
- Motivation variations
- Change in personality or behavioral patterns
- Withdrawal from companionship
- Decline in performance, both physically and academically
- Frequent missing of classes, especially physical activity classes
- Inability to coordinate (standing or walking)
- Poor personal hygiene and grooming
- Muddled speech
- Impaired judgment
- Restless, jittery
- Muscular twitches, tremor of hands
- Heavy sweating, bad breath, nervousness (amphetamine abuse)
- Red eyes, listlessness, increased appetite with special craving for sweets or salty foods (marijuana abuse)

Drug Education/Drug Testing

Through mandates by sport organizations, interscholastic, intercollegiate, amateur, and professional athletes are subject to anti-doping testing as it related to the use of prohibited substance and prohibited methods. This is an attempt to make the playing field as equal as possible for all participants. This has developed because performance enhancing drug use has become common at those levels. Another factor that has influenced this trend is the cost and reliability of drug tests. As with all issues of drug testing, the key is to educate the participants as to the detrimental effects of drug use. Most claims as to the beneficial effects of drug use are exaggerated. The best way to counter this is through proper education of the administrators, coaches, athletic trainers, athletes, and parents. Various organizations and groups have lists of banned, restricted and allowable substances. Please consult your local or state government or the sport governing body to clarify issues surrounding drug and supplement use. True Sport (www.truesport.org), an educational program designed by the United States Anti-Doping Agency, is available online and provided the learner a better understanding of quality offerings through sports participation.

Summary

Environmental issues must be clearly understood in order to avoid unnecessary injury and illness. Practice and competition can place the athlete under physical, mental, and emotional stress. Establishment and adherence to guidelines can help control the number of environmentally related incidents. Monitoring the weight gains and losses of individuals plus the adequate hydration of athletes is effective in the identification of individuals susceptible to environmental stress. Athletes are not immune to the various eating disorders commonly associated with our culture. Healthcare providers must be able to recognize that an athlete has a problem and provide that athlete with the proper referral. Eating disorders must be treated as any other physical illness/disease, should not be dismissed as a minor issue, and must be treated and monitored by a physician and other qualified health care providers. Knowledge of both legal and ethical issues will help the healthcare provider avoid unwarranted problems. Federal, state and local laws plus guidelines by national organizations provide the framework for healthcare professionals so work within those parameters. If your organization implements drug testing for athletes, develop a comprehensive written plan to protect everyone involved. The plan should contain the reasoning behind why there is a need to drug testing, random selection of athletes, who will handle test results, disciplinary action for positive drug test, and other associated costs.

References

Beals, K. (2004). *Disordered eating among athletes: A comprehensive guide for health professionals.* Champaign, IL: Human Kinetics.

Bergeron, M. (2002). Averting heat cramps. *Physician and Sports Medicine, 30*(11), p. 14.

Binkley, H., Beckett, J., Casa, D., Kleiner, D., & Plummer, P. (2002). National Athletic Trainers Association Position Statement: Exertional heat illnesses. *Journal of Athletic Training, 7*(3), pp. 329-342.

Binklet, H., Whitehill, W., Wright, K., & Dell-Pruett, M. (2009) The Drug Testing Process. *Strength & Conditioning Journal*, 31(6), 28-37.

Casa, D., Armstrong, L., Hillman, S., Mountain, S., & Reiff, R. (2002). National Athletic Trainers Association Position Statement: Fluid replacement for Athletes. *Journal of Athletic Training, 35*(2), pp. 212-242.

Center for Disease Control and Prevention. (April 2013) *Antibiotics Aren't Always the Answer.* Retrieved from http://www.cdc.gov/Features/GetSmart/.

Deere, R., & Wright, K. (2004). Health Insurance Portability and Accountability Act: Does It Affect You? *KAHPERD Journal, 40*(2).

France, R. (2004). *Introduction to sports medicine and athletic training.* New York, NY: Thomson Delmar Learning.

Gatorade Sports Science Institute. (2002). *Dehydration and heat illness: Identification, treatment, and prevention.* Chicago, IL: Gatorade Sports Science Institute.

Gatorade Sports Science Institute. (March 2013). Retrieved from www.gssi.com

Kohl, T., Martin, D., Nemeth, R., Evans, D., & Berks County Scholastic Athletic Trainers' Association(2000). *Wrestling Mats: Are they a Source of Ringworm Infection? Journal of Athletic Training, 35*(4).

Lohman, T. (1992). *Advances in body composition assessment.* Champaign, IL: Human Kinetics.

McArkle, W., Katch, W., & Katch, V. (2005). *Sports and exercise nutrition.* Philadelphia, PA: Lippincott, Williams, and Wilkins.

McArkle, W., Katch, F., & Katch, V., (1999). *Sports and exercise nutrition.* Philadelphia, PA: Lippincott, Williams, & Wilkins.

Moss, R. (2002). Another look at sudden death and exertional hyperthermia. *Athletic Therapy Today, 7*(3), pp. 44-45.

Nagel, D., Black, D., Leverenz, L., & Coster, D. (2000). Evaluation of a Screening Test for Female College Athletes with Eating Disorders and Disordered Eating. *Journal of Athletic Training, (35)*4.

National Federation of State High School Associations. (March 2013) *A Guide to Heat Acclimatization and Heat Illness Prevention.* Retrieved from www.nfhslearn.com.

National Athletic Trainers' Association Research and Education Foundation. (1997). *Dehydration and Heat Illness.* Dallas, TX: NATA Research & Education Foundation.

Porth, C. (1994). *Pathophysiology.* Philadelphia, PA: Lippincott.

Price, S., & Wilson, L. (1992). *Pathophysiology: Clinical concepts of disease processes.* St. Louis, MO: Mosby.

Sanborn, C. F. (2000). Disordered eating and the female athlete triad. *Clinicals in Sports Medicine, 19*(2), p. 199.

Sawyer, T. (2003). *A guide to sport nutrition: For student-athletes, coaches, athletic trainers, and parents.* Urbana, IL: Sagamore.

Sports, Cardiovascular, and Wellness Nutrition. (2013). Retrieved from www.scandpg.org

Taylor Hooton Foundation. (2013). Retrieved from www.taylorhooten.org

The National Center for Drug Free Sport. (2013). Retrieved from www.drugfreesport.com

United States Anti-Doping Agency. (2012). *Athlete handbook.* Retrieved from www.usada.org/athlete-handbook

United States Anti-Doping Agency. (2013). True sport. Retrieved from www.usada.org/truesport

United States Anti-Doping Agency. (2008). Targets Teens Addicted to Sports, Not Drugs. Retrieved from www.usada.org/ThatsDope.org

Walsh, K., Bennett, B., Cooper, M., & Holle, R. (2000). National Athletic Trainers Association Position Statement: Lightning safety for athletics and recreation. *Journal of Athletic Training, 35*(4), pp. 471-477.

Whitehill, W., Wright, K., & Deere, R. (2006). Doping in Sports: Seven Issues in Drug Testing. *KAHPERD Journal, 42*(2), pp. 26-29.

Wright, K. (1998). Pharmacology: Review for Athletic Training Educators. *Athletic Therapy Today,* Fall (3) 35-37.

Review Questions

Completion

1. The gradual process of adjusting to hot weather and cold weather workouts is known as _____. This process takes _____ weeks.

2. Frequent _____ _____ before, during, and after practice will help ensure that athletes function efficiently and safely..

3. A fluid loss of as little as _____ % of total body weight can adversely affect endurance and coordination.

4. _____ is a medical emergency.

5. Besides fluid replacement, two special concerns during cold weather workouts are _____ and _____.

6. The common cold virus is transmitted primarily by _____.

7. Pre-activity foods should exclude the following items:

8. The gender specific condition called "female triad" involves three components: _____, _____, and _____.

Short Answer

1. Why are high temperature and elevated humidity dangerous?

2. What factors cause heat stroke?

3. What are the symptoms of heat exhaustion?

4. What are the symptoms of heat stroke?

5. What are the first-aid procedures for heat stroke?

6. What are the progressive signs of hypothermia?

7. List three of the harmful side effects of steroid use.

8. What are some of the signs you should look for in substance use and abuse?

9. What can happen if an athlete returns to activity before fully recovering from a cold?

10. Define the differences between anorexia nervosa and bulimia.

Appendix A

Glossary

Base or Root Words

Term	Meaning	Term	Meaning
aden	gland	hystera	womb
angeion	vessel	ileum	small intestine
arteria	artery	iris	iris (of eye)
athron	joint	keras	cornea (of eye)
blepharon	eyelid	kinesis	movement
bronchos	bronchus	lac	milk
bursa	sac	larynx	throat
cardia	heart	mamma	breast
carpus	wrist	mastos	breast
cephale	head	meninx	membrane
chir	hand	mens	mind
chole	bile	mentra	womb
chondros	cartilage	mnesis	memory
coccyx	last spinal bone	musculus	muscle
colon	bowel	myelos	marrow
colpos	vagina	myo	muscle
core	pupil (of eye)	myringa	eardrum
corneus	cornea (of eye)	nephros	kidney
costa	rib	neuron	nerve
coax	hip	oophoros	ovary
cranium	skull	ophthalmos	eye
cutis	skin	opsis	sight
cystis	bladder	orchis	testicle
dacryon	tear	orexis	appetite
dactylos	finger	osme	smell
derma	skin	osteon	bone
diaphragma	diaphragm	otos	ear
dipsa	thirst	pathos	disease
emein	vomit	pectus	chest
enteron	gut	pes	foot
esophagus	gullet	pharynx	throat (part)
gala	milk	phases	speech
ganglion	nerve knot	philia	love
gaster	stomach	phlebos	vein
genos	origin	phobos	fear
glossa	tongue	phonos	voice
gone	gonad	phoreo	perspiration
hema	blood	plasso	formation
hepar	liver	plexis	stroke

pneumon	lung
podikos	foot
proktos	anus or rectum
psyche	mind
pyelos	kidney
pyloros	pelvis
ren	kidney
rhin	nose
salpinx	fallopian tube
sarx	flesh
sperma	semen
sphygmos	pulse
splen	spleen
stoma	mouth
tenon	tendon
thorax	chest
thymos	thymos
thyreos	thyroid
traches	windpipe
trichinos	hair
urina	urine
uterus	womb

Prefixes

Prefix	Meaning
a, an	without, lack of
ab	from, away from
ad	to
ambi	both
amphi	on both sides
ana	up, apart, across
ankylo	adhesion
ante, antero	before, in front
anti	against
apo	from
auto	self
bi	twice, double, two
bio	life
brachy	short
brady	slow
cata, kata	down
circum	around
co, com, con	with
contra	against, opposite
cyano	blue
cyto	cell
dactyl	finger, toe

Prefix	Meaning
de	away from
di	twice, double
dia	through
dis	apart from, not
dys	difficult, bad
e, ex	out of, out from
ecto	outer
em, en	in
endo	within
Prefix	Meaning
epi	on, upon
eso	inward
eu	good, well
exo	outside
extra	beyond, outside
hem, haem	blood
hemi	half
hetero	unlike
homo	similarity
hydro	water
hyper	over, above
hypo	less, under, below
im, in	in, not
infra	below
inter	between
intra	within
intro	into
iso	equal
kinesi	movement
leuco, leuko	white
macro	large
mal	ill, bad
megalo	great
melano	dark, black
meso	middle
meta	change, transformation
micro	small
multi	many
myo, my	muscle
neo	new
nephro	kidney
neuro	nerve
ob	in front of
oligo	few
ortho	straight
osteo	bone
pachy	thick

Prefix	Meaning	Prefix	Meaning
pan	all, every	quadri	four, four fold
para	beside	re	back again
per	through	retro	backward
peri	around	semi	half
platy	broad	sub	under, less than
pluri	several	sum, syn	with, together
polio	gray matter	super	above, more than
poly	many	supra	above, upon
post, poster	after, behind	tachy	fast
pre	before, in front	teno	tendon
pro	before, in behalf of	trans	through, across
proto	first	ultra	beyond, in excess
pesudo	false	uni	one
pyo	pus		

Anatomical Directions and Body Planes

Lateral and medial, superior and inferior are also used to indicate surfaces as well as directions or position.

ABDUCTION—movement away from the median plane around an anterior-posterior axis with the angle between the displaced parts becoming greater, as in lifting the arm sideward away from the body

ACTION—in physiology, the motions or functions of a part or organ of the body

ADDUCTION—movement toward the median plane around an anterior-posterior axis with the angle between the displaced parts becoming lesser, as in bringing the arm sideward against the body

ANATOMICAL POSITION—the neutral stance of the individual; standing, facing forward with arms at the sides and palms facing forward

ANTERIOR or VENTRAL—the front of the body or body part

CIRCUMDUCTION—is movement around the horizontal and longitudinal axis of a joint during which the distal end of the bone circumscribes the base of an imaginary cone and proximal end forms the apex, as in swinging the arms in a circle

DEPRESSION (down)—just the opposite, as in lowering the shoulder

DISTAL—farthest from a point of reference (opposite of proximal)

DORSIFLEXION—the act of drawing the toe or foot toward the dorsal aspect of the proximally conjoined body segment

DORSAL—upper surface (e.g., top of foot)

DORSUM—the back side of the hand

ELEVATION (up)—as in lifting the shoulder up

EVERSION—turning the sole of the foot outward

EXTENSION—is the reverse movement during which the angle between the anterior aspects of the displaced parts is increased as in moving the forearm away from the upper arm

EXTERNAL or PERIPHERAL—means near the surface

EXTERNAL ROTATION—turning outwardly or away from the midline of the body

FLEXION—movement around a transverse axis in an anterior-posterior plane with the angle between the anterior aspects of the displaced parts becoming smaller, as in bending the forearm toward the arm at the elbow joint

HYPER (prefix)—meaning too much

HYPEREXTENSION—in excess of normal extension

HYPERFLEXION—in excess of normal flexion

INFERIOR—toward the bottom of the body or body part

INSERTION—muscle attachment to a bone that moves

INTERNAL—refers to a deeper position

INTERNAL ROTATION—the turning of a limb toward the midline of the body

INVERSION—turning the sole of the foot inward

LATERAL—away from the midline of the body

MAJOR—Means greater or larger

MEDIAL—toward the midline of the body

MID SAGITTAL or MEDIAN—divides the body into equal and symmetrical right and left halves

MINOR—Means lesser or smaller

ORIGIN—the fixed end or attachment of muscle

PALMAR—ventral aspect of the hand (palm of the hand)

PLANTAR—ventral aspect of the foot (sole of the foot)

PLANTAR FLEXION—the act of drawing the toe or foot toward the plantar aspect of the proximally conjoined body segment

POSTERIOR or DORSAL—the back of the body or body part

PRONATION—is medial rotation of the forearm, as in turning the palm of the hand downward

PRONE—face down, horizontal position of the body

PROTRACTION—(forward) as in bring the shoulder forward

PROXIMAL—nearest to the point of attachment, origin or other point of reference

RANGE OF MOTION (ROM)—The extent to which a body part can move through all of its planes of movement

RETRACTION (backward)—as in pulling the shoulder back and thus bringing the shoulder blades together

ROTATION—is movement around a longitudinal axis which passes through a joint as in turning the palm of the hand up or down with the arm abducted

SUPERFICIAL—toward the surface of the body

SUPERIOR—toward the top of the body or body part

SUPINATION—is lateral rotation of the forearm, as in turning the palm of the hand upward

SUPINE—lying on the back, face upward, opposed to prone

VALGUS—position of a body part that is bent outward

VARUS—position of a body part that is bent inward

VENTRAL—bottom surface (opposite of dorsal)

VOLAR—ventral aspect of the hand

Anatomical Structures

ACROMIOCLAVICULAR JOINT—Joint formed by the distal clavicle and the acromion process of the scapula

ANATOMICAL SNUFF BOX—The space at the base of the thumb created by the extensor pollicis longus and brevis tendons

ANTERIOR CRUCIATE LIGAMENT—A ligament crossing through the knee joint that attaches from the anterior tibia to the posterior femur. It limits anterior movement of the tibia from the femur as well as rotation of the tibia

ARTICULAR SURFACES—The ends of bones which move on each other. These surfaces are covered with a thin layer of cartilage (hyaline cartilage) to ensure smooth movement

APPENDICULAR SKELETON—consists of the bones of the shoulder and the upper extremities, and the hips and the lower extremities. These bones form the appendages and attach to the axial skeleton

ARTICULATION—a joint between bones; The manner of connecting by a joint

AXIAL SKELETON—composed of the bones of the skull, the thorax, and the vertebral column. These bones form the axis of the body

AXILLA—arm pit

BICEPS—muscle on front of upper arm

BONE—a supportive rigid connective tissue consisting of an abundant calcified matrix enclosing many branched cells

BURSA—a fluid-filled sac or saclike cavity that allows a muscle or tendon to slide over bone (thereby eliminating friction). [BURSAE—plural]

CALCANEOUS—heel bone

CARTILAGE—a connective tissue characterized by its nonvascularity and firm consistency

CERVICAL—of the neck, especially the seven vertebrae in the neck

CHONDRAL—pertaining to cartilage

COCCYX—the four rudimentary bones at lowest end of the backbone; the vestigial human tail

COSTOCHONDRAL—rib and its cartilage

CRANIAL—of, or pertaining to the skull or superior part of the body, opposed to caudal

CRUCIATE—cross shaped

CUBITAL FOSSA—triangular area on the anterior aspect of the forearm directly opposite the elbow joint (the bend of the elbow)

CUTANEOUS—skin

DERMATOME—segmental skin area innervated by various spinal cord segments

DERMAL—pertaining to the dermis; cutaneous

DIARTHRODIAL JOINT—a ball and socket joint

DIGIT—finger/toe

EPIPHYSIS—growth plate

FASCIA—fibrous membrane that covers, supports, and separates muscles

HAMSTRINGS—a muscle group in the posterior thigh consisting of the semitendinosus, semimembranosus, and biceps femoris

HYPOTHENAR EMINENCE—Intrinsic muscles of the thumb

ILIAC CREST—the superior border of the iliac bone; a contusion to this area is called a "hip pointer"

JOINT CAPSULE, ARTICULAR CAPSULE, SYNOVIAL CAPSULE—a saclike, fibrous membrane that surrounds a joint.; Often including or interwoven with ligaments

LIGAMENT—a band of flexible, tough, dense white fibrous connective tissue connecting the articular ends of the bones and sometimes enveloping them in a capsule

LONGITUDINAL ARCH—from heel to toes on the under surface of the foot

LUMBAR—vertebral column extending from the twentieth through the twenty-fourth vertebrae; Low back

MALLEOLUS—a rounded bony protuberance on each side of the ankle joint

MENISCI—curved fibrocartilages used to deepen the articular facets of the knee

MENISCUS—in anatomy, a crescent-shaped structure, serving to adapt the articular surfaces to one another

MUSCLE—a tissue composed of contractile fibers or cells. A contractile organ composed of muscle tissue, affecting the movements of the organs and parts of the body

NERVE—a bundle of nerve fibers, usually outside the brain or spinal cord

PHALANGES—bones of the fingers or toes

PLANTAR FASCIA—tough bands of tissue on the sole of the foot

POPLITEAL SPACE—area behind the knee joint

QUADRICEPS—the muscle group in the anterior thigh consisting of the rectus femoris, vastus medialis, vastus intermedius, and vastus lateralis

ROTATOR CUFF—the muscle group in the shoulder consisting of the subscapularis, supraspinatus, infraspinatus, and teres minor

SESAMOID BONE—a small bone implanted in a tendon

TENDON—a band of dense fibrous tissue forming the termination of a muscle and attaching to a bone

THORACIC—portion of vertebral column extending from the eighth through the nineteenth vertebrae; mid/upper back

THENAR EMINENCE—intrinsic muscles of the thumb that include the abductor pollicis brevis, flexor pollicis brevis, opponens pollicis, and adductor pollicis

Classifications of Injuries

ACUTE—quick onset, short duration

ADHESION—a sticking together or binding of tissue fibers

ANTISEPTIC—a substance which prevents the growth of bacteria

AVASCULAR—Without blood or lymphatic vessels. This may be a normal state as in certain forms of cartilage, or as a result of disease or injury

BENIGN—Harmless

BUNIONETTE—bony enlargement of lateral side of the head of 5th metatarsal at the metatarsophalangeal joint; associated with an overlying bursa sac and a medial deviation of the 5th phalange

BURSITIS—inflammation of a bursa

CHRONDROMALACIA—softening of a cartilage

CHRONIC—of long duration, repeating; In athletes, usually a injury that has not responded to treatment

CONGENITAL—existing before or at birth; Dating from, but not necessarily detected at birth

CONTUSION—a bruise; an injury usually caused by a blow in which the skin is not broken

CREPITUS—grating sound produced by the contact of the fractured ends of bones

DIAGNOSIS (or Evaluation)—the determination of the nature of an injury or disease

DISLOCATION—the displacement of one or more bones of a joint, or of any organ from the original position

ECCHYMOSIS—extravasation (escape into tissues) of blood; also the tissue discoloration caused by the extravasation of blood

EDEMA—swelling as a result of the collection of fluid in the connective tissue

EFFUSION—escape of the fluid into a cavity

EPISTAXIS—nosebleed

EXOSTOSIS—a benign cartilage; capped protuberance from the surface of long bones, but also seen on flat bones; due to chronic irritation as from infection, trauma, or osteoarthritis

FASCIITIS—inflammation of fascia

FRACTURE—the breaking of a bone or cartilage

HEMATOMA—a circumscribed extravascular collection of blood, usually clotted, which forms a mass

HEMATURIA—passing of blood in the urine

HEMORRHAGE—escaping of blood through ruptured walls of vessels

HERNIA—the abnormal protrusion of an organ, or a part, through the containing wall of its cavity, usually the abdominal cavity, beyond its normal confines

INFLAMMATION—reaction of the body tissue to an irritant

JOINT SUBLUXATION—partial displacement of the articular surfaces and crepitus; there is a first- or second-degree ligamentous injury

LACERATION—a tear, or a wound made by tearing; the act of tearing or lacerating

MYOSITIS OSSIFICANS—inflammation of muscle, with formation of bone

MYOSITIS—inflammation of muscle tissue

NECROSIS—Death of tissue or cells

OPEN WOUND—a wound or injury involving a break in the skin

OSGOOD SCHLATTERS—osteochondrosis of the tuberosity of the tibia, seen especially in adolescents (Inflammation of both bone and cartilage)

OSTEOCHONDRITIS DISSECANS—a joint characterized by partial or complete detachment of a fragment or articular cartilage and underlying bone

PARALYSIS—loss of power of voluntary motion

PLANTAR FASCIITIS—inflammation at origin of plantar fascia

SEPARATION—injury to a non-movable joint

SPRAIN—a wrenching of a joint, producing a stretching or tearing of the ligaments

SPUR—an outgrowth of bony tissue into muscles or skin

STRAIN—excessive stretching or overuse of a part, as of tendon/muscle

SUBACUTE—relatively acute; a stage between acute and chronic; after the initial trauma

SUBLUXATION—partial displacement of the articular surfaces

SYNDROME—group of typical symptoms or conditions that characterize a deficiency or disease

TENDINITIS—inflammation of a tendon or musculoskeletal junction

TENOSYNOVITIS—inflammation of a tendon and its sheath

TRAUMA—wound or injury

Terms: Taping and Wrapping

ANCHOR—anything that makes stable or secure, anything that is depended upon for support or security

BUTTERFLY—strips of tape that overlaps, as in "X" pattern

CAST—to produce a specific form by pouring material (metal, plaster, etc.) into a prepared mold

CHECK REIN—reinforced tape to prevent movement

COLLATERAL—meaning side, lateral and medial

COMPRESSION—the act of applying pressure to an organ (i.e., applying a wrap, beginning at the bottom of an injury and wrapping towards the heart)

DIAGONALLY—a slanted or oblique direction

DIAMOND SHAPE—an object that is in the shape of two equilateral triangles placed base to base

EXTENSION WRAP—a wrap used to assist in the extension of a specific joint

FIGURE OF EIGHT—the bandaging of a joint where the initial turn circles the one part of the joint and the second turn circles the adjoining part of the joint to form a figure of eight

FLEXION WRAP—a wrap used to assist in the flexion of that joint

HORIZONTAL STRIP—a strip that is placed level with the horizon, opposed to vertical strip

HORSESHOE—padding made to resemble the "U" shape

HOT SPOT—Early redness of the skin from friction that leads to a blister formation if preventive measures are not taken

MUSCLE CONTRACTED—the shortening of the muscle

PRICES (acronym)—Protection, Rest, Ice, Compression, Elevation, and Support

PAD SUPPORT—a pad placed in a certain area to sustain, hold up, or maintain a desired position

PROPHYLACTIC—Denoting something that is preventative or protective

SHORTEN THE ANGLE OF PULL—decreasing the range of motion of a joint

SPICA WRAP—a figure eight bandage that generally overlaps the previous to form V like designs; used to give support, apply pressure or hold a dressing

SPIRAL—applying a bandage around a limb that ascends the body part overlapping the previous bandage

STIRRUP—Any "U" shaped loop or piece

SUPPORT—to sustain, hold up or maintain a desired position

SWELLING—an increase in size of an area due to an increase in fluid

TAPE MASS—adhesive applied to the cloth comprised of natural synthetic, zinc oxide, etc.

VERTICAL STRIP—a strip that is placed perpendicular to the line of the horizon, opposed to horizontal strip

X-PATTERN—the crossing of two pieces of tape in the shape of an X

Appendix B

Websites for Health Care and Sport Industry Professionals

American Academy of Dermatology www.aad.org
American Academy of Family Physicians www.aafp.org
American Academy of Neurology www.aan.com
American Academy of Ophthalmology www.aao.org
American Academy of Orthopaedic Surgeons www.aaos.org
American Academy of Otolaryngology www.entnet.org
American Academy of Pain Management www.aapainmanage.org
American Academy of Pediatrics (AAP) www.aap.org
American Academy of Podiatric Sports Medicine (AAPSM) www.aapsm.org
American Academy of Physical Medicine and Rehabilitation (AAPMR) www.aapmr.org
American Chiropractic Association www.acasc.org
American College of Foot and Ankle Surgeons www.acfas.org
American College of Sports Medicine www.acsm.org
American Dental Association www.ada.org
American Dietetic Association www.eatright.org
American Heart Association www.americanheart.org
American Kinesiotherapy Association www.akta.org
American Massage Therapy Association www.amtamassage.org
American Medical Association www.ama-assn.org
American Medical Society for Sport Medicine www.amssm.org
American Occupational Therapy Association www.aota.org
American Optometric Association www.aoa.org
American Orthopaedic Foot and Ankle Society www.aofas.org
American Orthopaedic Society for Sports Medicine www.sportsmed.org
American Osteopathic Academy of Sport Medicine www.aoasm.org
American Osteopathic Association www.osteopathic.org
American Physical Therapy Association (APTA) www.apta.org
American Physical Therapy Association Sports Physical Therapy Section www.spts.org
American Alliance for Health, Physical Education, Recreation and Dance www.aahperd.org
American Association for Physical Activity and Recreation (AAPAR) www.aapar.org
America's Health Insurance Plan www.hiaa.org
American Red Cross *www.redcross.org*
American Red Cross – Athletic Training Education Competencies *www.redcross.org/AthleticTrainers*
American Sports Medicine Institute *www.asmi.org*
Athlete Performance Institute *www.athletesperformance.com*
Andrews Institute *www.theandrewsinstitute.com/*
Academy for Sports Dentistry (ASD) *www.academyforsportsdentistry.org*
Association for Applied Sport Psychology *www.appliedsportpsych.org*
Association for Sports Medicine in Industry, Business and Military *www.theindustrialathlete.com*
Association of Sport Performance Centres *http://forumelitesport.org*
Canadian Academy of Sport & Exercise Medicine *www.casem-acmse.org*
Canadian Athletic Therapists Association *www.athletictherapy.org*
Canadian Centre for Ethics in Sports *www.cces.ca*
Centers for Disease Control and Prevention *www.cdc.gov*
College Athletic Trainers' Society *www.collegeathletictrainer.org*
Collegiate Strength and Conditioning Coaches *www.cscca.org*
Collegiate & Professional Sport Dietitians Association (CPSDA) *www.sportrd.org*
Disney Sports Attraction *http://espnwwos.disney.go.com*

Drug Free Sport *www.drugfreesport.com*
Food and Nutrition Information Center *www.nalusda.gov/fnic*
Gatorade Sports Science Institute *www.gssiweb.com*
HealthSouth *www.healthsouth.com*
Hughston Orthopaedic and Sports Medicine *www.hughston.com*
IMG Academy *www.imgacademy.com*
Industrial Athlete Institute for Research and Education (IAIRE) *www.theindustrialathlete.com*
International Olympic Committee *www.olympic.org*
International Society for Sports Psychiatry (ISSP) *www.SportsPsychiatry.org*
Joint Commission on Sports Medicine and Science *www.jcsportsmedicine.org*
Joseph Institute for Ethics *www.charactercounts.org*
Mayo Clinic *www.mayoclinic.org*
National Athletic Trainers' Association *www.nata.org*
National Athletic Trainers' Association Board of Certification *www.bocatc.org*
National Association for Sport and Physical Education *www.aahperd.org/naspe*
National Center for Drug Free Sports *www.drugfreesport.com*
National Center for Sports Safety *www.SportsSafety.org*
National Collegiate Athletic Association *www.ncaa.org*
National Federation of State High School Athletic Associations (NFHS) *www.nfhs.org*
NFHS Coach Education *www.nfhslearn.com*
National Interscholastic Athletic Administrators Association *www.niaaa.org*
National Institutes of Health *www.nih.gov*
National Lightning Safety Institute *www.lightningsafety.com*
National Operating Committee on Standards for Athletic Equipment (NOCSEA) *www.nocsae.org*
National Strength and Conditioning Association (NSCA) *www.nsca.com*
National Safety Council *www.nsc.org*
North American Society for Pediatric Exercise Medicine (NASPEM) *www.naspem.org*
Occupational Safety and Health Administration (OSHA) *www.osha.gov*
President's Council on Fitness, Sports, and Nutrition (PCFSN) *www.presidentschallenge.org*
Special Olympics International *www.specialolympics.org*
Sports, Cardiovascular and Wellness Nutrition (SCAN) *www.scandpg.org*
Sport Information Resource Centre (SIRC) *www.sirc.ca*
Stop Sports Injuries *www.STOPSortsInjuries.org*
Taylor Hooten Foundation *www.taylorhooten.org*
United States Anti-Doping Agency (USADA) *www.usantidoping.org*
United States Olympic Committee (USOC) *www.usolympicteam.com*
World Anti-Doping Agency *www.wada-ama.org*

Index

Instructions for

Online Material Access

Steps to redeem access code if you DO NOT currently have a Sagamore Account

1. Go to **http://www.sagamorepub.com.**

2. Click on the **register** link and fill out the requested information.

3. Enter the code provided at the end of this book in the **online access code field.**

4. Click on **Create New Account.**

5. Click on **My Materials** tab to access all additional materials provided with your book purchase.

Steps to Redeem Code if you currently DO HAVE a Sagamore Account

1. Go to **http://www.sagamorepub.com.**

2. Click on the **Login** link and proceed to login.

3. Click on the **Access Codes tab** for your account, enter the code provided at the end of this book and click Submit.

4. Click on the **My Materials** tab to access all additional materials provided with your book purchase.

If you have any questions, please select the contact us tab at www.sagamorepub.com

Online Materials Access Code

BAT6-6WHG0KRQD2WE

Comprehensive Manual of Taping, Wrapping, and Protective Devices

4th Edition

Recognized as the comprehensive text in athletic taping and wrapping techniques for healthcare professionals, the fourth edition of the *Comprehensive Manual of Taping, Wrapping, and Protective Devices* has been enhanced by the addition of selected audio and video segments, kinesio taping techniques, and a visual display of protective devices. Written by recognized experts in sport medicine, this text displays and describes a step-by-step process in the application of taping and wrapping products along with a listing of protective devices to be utilized in preventing injuries. The *Comprehensive Manual of Taping, Wrapping, and Protective Devices* will feature online supplements along with instructor resources.

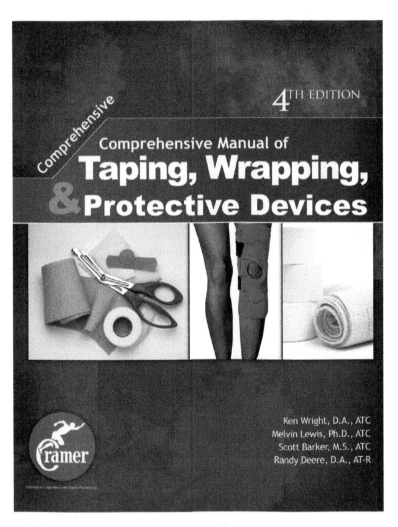